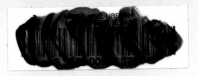

THE EVERYTHING®
LOW-CARB MEAL PREP COOKBOOK

Dear Reader,

If you're reading this, that means you've decided not only to take the plunge into a low-carbohydrate diet, but also to try your hand at meal prep. Bravo, my friend. Your life is about to change for the better.

Low-carbohydrate diets have been around since the 1800s, but they didn't gain a lot of attention until the 1990s when the Atkins diet became popular. Even as low-carbohydrate diets made their way into the mainstream, laypeople and nutrition professionals alike were scoffing at the idea, calling it a fad diet and insisting that the trend was unhealthy. Well, not so fast. Since 2002, there have been over two dozen human studies done on low-carbohydrate diets, and in each one of these studies, the low-carbohydrate diets proved superior to their competitors. Participants not only saw an increase in weight loss, they also presented with reduced markers for diabetes and heart disease.

When you add the power of the low-carb diet to the concept of meal prepping, you score a double win for your health. In this book, you'll find 300 simple, low-carbohydrate recipes, and every single one is designed to provide you with at least six servings. You can follow the same meal plan for six days in a row and enjoy these meals all week, or in some cases, you can freeze them and save them for later. That part is totally up to you. There are also sample menu plans that I've created to make life even easier for you. You can utilize these as you get the hang of meal planning and then create your own meal plans once you're a seasoned pro.

However you decide to use this book, I hope that you find the information enlightening and that the low-carb recipes become a regular part of your meal prep routine. I wish you all the best.

Lindsay Boyers, CHNC

Oct 18

Welcome to the EVERYTHING® Series!

These handy, accessible books give you all you need to tackle a difficult project, gain a new hobby, comprehend a fascinating topic, prepare for an exam, or even brush up on something you learned back in school but have since forgotten.

You can choose to read an Everything® book from cover to cover or just pick out the information you want from our four useful boxes: e-questions, e-facts, e-alerts, and e-ssentials. We give you everything you need to know on the subject, but throw in a lot of fun stuff along the way too.

We now have more than 400 Everything® books in print, spanning such wide-ranging categories as weddings, pregnancy, cooking, music instruction, foreign language, crafts, pets, New Age, and so much more. When you're done reading them all, you can finally say you know Everything®!

QUESTION

Answers to common questions

FACT

Important snippets of information

ALERT

Urgent warnings

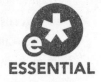

ESSENTIAL

Quick handy tips

PUBLISHER Karen Cooper

MANAGING EDITOR Lisa Laing

COPY CHIEF Casey Ebert

ASSOCIATE PRODUCTION EDITOR Jo-Anne Duhamel

ACQUISITIONS EDITOR Zander Hatch

SENIOR DEVELOPMENT EDITOR Brett Palana-Shanahan

EVERYTHING® SERIES COVER DESIGNER Erin Alexander

Visit the entire Everything® series at www.everything.com

THE EVERYTHING® Low-Carb Meal Prep Cookbook

Lindsay Boyers, CHNC

Adams Media
New York London Toronto Sydney New Delhi

To the late Mr. Lindsey, my middle school English teacher at St. Theresa School, who made sure we were reading and writing at a high school level by the sixth grade. Thank you for giving me the skills that led me on the path to becoming a writer. Every time I'm accused of being a "grammar nerd," I think of you fondly.

To Janet Schwartz, my nutrition professor at Framingham State University and current chair of the food and nutrition department, who told me I should be a writer after reading one of my assignments. Those five words had more impact than you realized. Thank you.

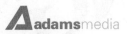

Adams Media
An Imprint of Simon & Schuster, Inc.
57 Littlefield Street
Avon, Massachusetts 02322

An Everything® Series Book.
Everything® and everything.com® are registered trademarks of Simon & Schuster, Inc.

First Adams Media trade paperback edition August 2018

ADAMS MEDIA and colophon are trademarks of Simon & Schuster.

For information about special discounts for bulk purchases, please contact Simon & Schuster Special Sales at 1-866-506-1949 or business@ simonandschuster.com.

The Simon & Schuster Speakers Bureau can bring authors to your live event. For more information or to book an event contact the Simon & Schuster Speakers Bureau at 1-866-248-3049 or visit our website at www.simonspeakers.com.

Photographs by James Stefiuk

Manufactured in the United States of America

10 9 8 7 6 5 4 3 2 1

Library of Congress Cataloging-in-Publication Data
Boyers, Lindsay, author.
The everything low-carb meal prep cookbook / Lindsay Boyers, CHNC.
Avon, Massachusetts: Adams Media, 2018.
Series: Everything.
Includes index. .
LCCN 2018011468 | ISBN 9781507207314 (pb) | ISBN 9781507207321 (ebook)
LCSH: Low-carbohydrate diet--Recipes.
| BISAC: COOKING / Health & Healing / Low Carbohydrate. | COOKING / Methods / Quantity. | HEALTH & FITNESS / Diets. | LCGFT: Cookbooks.
LCC RM237.73 .B69 2018 | DDC 641.5/6383--dc23
LC record available at https://lccn.loc .gov/2018011468

ISBN 978-1-5072-0731-4
ISBN 978-1-5072-0732-1 (ebook)

Contents

Acknowledgments

Thank you to my family for always supporting me no matter what I'm doing. I don't know how I would do anything without you. I love you.

Thank you to anyone who has ever taken the time to read anything I've written. You keep me going. I hope you find some life-changing information along the way.

Introduction

ON ITS OWN, A low-carbohydrate diet is extremely powerful. It can help boost weight loss, reduce LDL cholesterol and triglyceride levels, get your blood sugar in check, and (arguably the best part) actually keep you feeling full and satiated. When you combine a low-carbohydrate diet with meal prep, you become a force to be reckoned with. You not only get all the health benefits of the low-carbohydrate diet, but you also get the added perk of always having a home-cooked, nutritionally balanced meal at your fingertips.

Meal prep—or planning out and cooking (or freezing) your meals in advance—is vital to your success on any diet. If you're not prepared, you are less likely to succeed. Meal prepping not only keeps you on track, it also helps save time and money, reduces stress, and ensures that your diet is nutritionally balanced. No more skipping meals because you're unprepared!

In this book, you'll find 300 simple, low-carbohydrate recipes, and each one is designed to provide you with at least six servings. You can follow the same meal plan for six days in a row and enjoy these meals all week, or in some cases, you can freeze them and save them for later. You choose the option that is most convenient for your life. You'll also find sample menu plans to make life even easier for you. You can utilize these as you get the hang of meal planning and then create your own meal plans once you're a seasoned pro.

The key to meal prep success is planning ahead: taking some time out of your week to sit down and write out exactly what you're going to be eating (and when) for the entire week. If you're consistent with this practice week after week, eventually two things will happen. You will reach (and surpass) your goal—whether it's weight loss, a reduction in blood pressure, more energy, or just a healthier lifestyle—and meal prepping will become such a regular part of your routine that you won't even have to think twice about it.

They say it takes twenty-one days to build a consistent habit, so why not start there? Make a commitment to stay on your low-carb diet for twenty-one days and to have every one of your meals for those twenty-one days prepped and ready to go. If you make this commitment to yourself and you stick with it, your life will change for the better. You'll quickly experience the benefits of a healthy eating routine, such as feeling better, sleeping better, and having higher levels of energy. Before you know it, meal prepping will become an essential tool for living your healthiest and best life!

CHAPTER 1

Low-Carb Diet Basics

Research shows that one of the most common reasons people are unsuccessful on any diet plan is a lack of preparation. Even with the best of intentions, if you don't plan ahead, you'll have a hard time reaching your goals. One of the best things about a low-carb diet is that it's designed to keep your hunger steady, so if you follow the diet plan as designed and make sure you always have a low-carb meal ready at your fingertips, you'll greatly increase your chances of success.

Breaking Down the Low-Carb Diet

Low-carb diet is a general term that implies a reduction in carbohydrates. Different low-carb diets have varying guidelines on how many carbohydrates, proteins, and fats you should eat daily, so they're not all the same, but typically, a low-carb diet macronutrient breakdown looks something like this:

- Less than 20 percent of calories from carbohydrates
- 25–30 percent of calories from protein
- 50–55 percent of calories from fat

QUESTION

How many grams of carbohydrates should I eat per day?
There is no set rule when it comes to how many grams of carbohydrates you should eat on a low-carb diet, but most people fall in the range of 25–150 grams per day, depending on their age, gender, activity level, and calorie needs.

Most low-carb diets eliminate the obvious sources of carbohydrates, like sugar, processed foods, and desserts—foods that are beneficial to eliminate for many reasons other than just their high carbohydrate count. Others eliminate fruit and starchy vegetables like potatoes, while some allow small amounts. There is no one-size-fits-all low-carb diet; it's up to you to find the balance of macronutrients and food choices that works for your body.

Total Carbs versus Net Carbs

When following a low-carb diet, you're likely to see or hear the term *net carbs.* This term, which is used to differentiate among types of carbohydrates, was developed by food manufacturers when the low-carb diet became really popular. The concept of net carbs is that certain carbohydrates affect your body in different ways, so you can count them differently when following a low-carb diet.

Refined sugars and starches—or carbohydrates that come from things like potatoes, white bread, and sugar-laden desserts—are absorbed quickly into your bloodstream, thus causing a rapid spike in blood sugar and insulin and affecting the way your body stores fat. On the other hand, complex carbohydrates—like the fiber from fruits and vegetables—move slowly through the digestive system and have little to no effect on blood sugar and insulin levels. In fact, some carbohydrates like insoluble fiber and sugar alcohols (erythritol and xylitol, to name a couple) move through the digestive system without entering your blood at all.

Based on this concept, some low-carb diets require you to count net carbohydrates instead of total carbohydrates. To calculate net carbohydrates, you simply subtract fiber and sugar alcohols from the total carbohydrate count. For example, if food contains 10 grams of total carbohydrates but 5 of those carbohydrates come from fiber and 1 comes from sugar alcohols, then the net carbs would be 4 grams.

The Difference Between Low-Carb and Ketogenic

People often use the terms *low-carb diet* and *ketogenic diet* interchangeably, but the two diets differ significantly. By definition, a low-carb diet is one that restricts carbohydrates but allows moderate amounts of both protein and fat. A ketogenic diet severely limits carbohydrates, sometimes down to 5–10 percent of calories, and limits protein as well. Fat makes up the bulk of a ketogenic diet, and the macronutrient breakdown typically looks like this:

- 5–10 percent of calories from carbohydrates
- 15–30 percent of calories from protein
- 60–75 percent of calories from fat

The goal of a ketogenic diet is to kick your body into ketosis—a state in which the body uses ketones, which are by-products of fat metabolism, instead of glucose for energy. On a standard low-carb diet, you may or may not enter a state of ketosis, but that's not the major goal.

ALERT

On a ketogenic diet, carbohydrates are typically limited to 50 grams or less per day. Ketogenic diets require you to count carbohydrates more diligently than low-carb diets because eating too many carbohydrates will throw you out of ketosis.

The Benefits of a Low-Carb Diet

Before diving into the how and why of meal planning, it's helpful to know all the benefits of low-carb diets. Of course, weight loss is a big one, but low-carb diets offer significant health benefits beyond weight loss alone. When you understand the mechanisms of how something affects your body positively, you're more likely to stay on track.

Weight Loss

Low-carb diets help you shed extra pounds fairly quickly. This works in two major ways. When you reduce your carbohydrate intake, your insulin levels decrease. In the initial stages of the diet, this drop in insulin prompts your kidneys, which are responsible for maintaining electrolyte balance, to release excess sodium. As sodium is released, the body also releases the extra water it was holding to keep the sodium properly diluted. As a result, you may experience a significant reduction in water weight, especially in the first two weeks.

QUESTION

Isn't water weight loss temporary?
Water weight fluctuates all the time. What you're eating, how much water you're drinking, and your hormonal cycles all affect how much water you're retaining on a daily basis. The loss of water weight in the initial stages of the low-carb diet is a great motivator because it leaves you feeling slimmer and less bloated, but to experience true fat loss, you have to stick to your low-carb diet for the long term.

The longer-term weight loss benefit of a low-carb diet is fat loss. There are two major types of fat in the body: subcutaneous fat and visceral fat. Subcutaneous fat lies just below the surface of your skin. It's the type of fat that's measured when doing body fat analysis and the type of fat that's responsible for cellulite. About 80 percent of the fat on your body is subcutaneous fat. The other type of fat is called visceral fat. Visceral fat lies deeper in your body and wraps around the inner organs in your abdomen. Visceral fat is significantly more dangerous than subcutaneous fat. Visceral fat drives inflammation, which increases your risk of diabetes, heart disease, stroke, and dementia. Studies show that low-carb diets not only result in more over-all fat loss than low-fat diets, but they also contribute to a greater reduction in visceral fat, specifically.

ALERT

If you hold most of your excess weight in your belly, it's a good indica-tion that you have too much visceral fat. Women with a waist circum-ference of more than thirty-five inches and men with a waist circumfer-ence of more than forty inches are at the greatest risk of developing the serious diseases associated with visceral fat.

Another way that low-carb diets contribute to weight loss is by balancing your hunger hormones. There are three major hormones involved in appe-tite regulation and fat storage: ghrelin, leptin, and insulin.

Ghrelin makes you feel hungry. When ghrelin is released into your blood from your stomach, it sends signals to the brain that trigger your appe-tite. Levels typically rise before meals and lower after meals. Ghrelin also promotes fat storage. Leptin does the opposite of ghrelin. When leptin is released from your fat cells, it sends signals to the brain that you're full and you should stop eating.

Research done by Dr. David Cummings of the University of Washington School of Medicine shows that when it comes to your diet, it's not calories that affect the levels of ghrelin and leptin in your blood, it's the macronutrients—carbohydrates, protein, and fat. During Dr. Cummings's research, he found that while eating carbohydrates initially lowered your levels of ghrelin and increased leptin, after a short time, the opposite occurred. Ghrelin came back with a vengeance, and leptin decreased significantly. As a result, participants experienced appetites that were even stronger than before the carbohydrate-rich meal.

On the other hand, protein showed the opposite effect. Participants who ate high-protein, low-carb meals experienced lowered ghrelin levels and increased leptin levels that stayed that way long after their meals were gone. In addition, the high-protein meals slowed the emptying of the stomach, helping participants feel full for a longer period of time.

The consumption of fat had a somewhat intermediate effect on ghre-lin and leptin. The takeaway message: eating fat doesn't cause the same decrease and subsequent increase as carbohydrates, but it doesn't keep you full as long as protein.

FACT

Research also shows that a lack of sleep negatively affects ghrelin and leptin levels. One study done at the University of Chicago reported that men who slept for four hours per night had ghrelin levels that were 28 percent higher and leptin levels that were 18 percent lower than those who slept ten hours. When trying to lose weight and control your hunger, consider your sleeping schedule as well. Are you getting enough?

Better Blood Sugar/Insulin Control

Low-carb diets also have a significant effect on insulin, a hormone that controls blood sugar levels and affects hunger as well. When you eat carbohydrates they are broken down into a simple sugar called glucose in your digestive tract. Glucose moves from your digestive tract into your bloodstream, where it triggers your pancreas to release the hormone insulin. Insulin attaches to the glucose molecules and carries them to your cells, where they're either used immediately for energy or stored for later use.

In a healthy person with a normal insulin response, this cascade of events normalizes blood sugar levels; however, it's estimated that in the United States alone, there are 60–70 million people whose bodies don't respond to insulin in a healthy way. This condition is called insulin resistance.

In people with insulin resistance, the cells of the muscle, fat, and liver don't respond properly to insulin, causing a negative cascade of events. When insulin can't bring the glucose from the blood into the cells, it triggers the pancreas to produce more insulin, putting pressure on the beta cells. In the early stages of insulin resistance, this increase in insulin is enough to get glucose out of the blood and into the body's cells; however, over time the beta cells in the pancreas cannot keep up with the body's demand for more insulin. The beta cells start to malfunction, and the pancreas becomes unable to produce insulin. If this condition is not corrected, it can lead to pre-diabetes, diabetes, and their resulting complications, such as heart disease, stroke, and loss of kidney function.

When you follow a low-carb diet, your blood glucose levels don't increase as significantly, also eliminating the need for excess amounts of insulin. As a result, both your blood sugar and insulin levels remain on an even keel, taking pressure off your pancreas and allowing your body to run more efficiently. In one study published in the scientific journal *Nutrition & Metabolism*, 95.2 percent of diabetic participants who followed a low-carb diet for six months were able to reduce or completely eliminate their need for diabetes medications.

FACT

If you have diabetes, talk to your doctor before going on a low-carb diet. Do not adjust your medication or insulin dosages without clearance from your health team and proper medical supervision.

Heart Benefits

In addition to the positive effects on blood sugar and hormone levels, low-carb diets have also been shown to improve all the significant markers for heart disease: low-density lipoprotein (or LDL), high-density lipoprotein (or HDL), triglycerides, and blood pressure.

Cholesterol in itself is not a bad thing. In fact, it's absolutely vital to your survival. Your body uses cholesterol to make vitamin D and certain very important hormones like estrogen, testosterone, cortisol, and DHEA, to name a few. People typically refer to LDL and HDL as bad cholesterol and good cholesterol, respectively, but each is somewhat of a misnomer. LDL and HDL are not actually cholesterol but rather proteins that carry cholesterol around in the blood. LDL carries cholesterol from the liver where it's made to the rest of the body, while HDL removes cholesterol from the artery walls and brings it back to the liver where it can be reused or excreted from the body. In a standard test, if your LDL is high, that's "bad," and if your HDL is high, that's "good," but unfortunately, it's not that simple.

More important than the number of LDL and HDL floating around in your blood is the size of the cholesterol particles. Small, dense LDL particles, also called lipoprotein(a) or Lp(a), cause inflammation of the blood and make it "sticky." The inflammation combined with the stickiness is what causes plaque buildup and makes you more susceptible to blood clotting, heart attack, and stroke. The more Lp(a) particles you have in your blood, the more likely you are to develop cardiovascular disease; however, you could have a normal LDL level according to standardized tests, but if all those LDL particles are Lp(a), you have a problem.

Research has shown that low-carb diets not only reduce the total number of LDL particles floating around in the blood, but they can actually change the size of the LDL particles, turning the small, dense particles into large, fluffy particles, which don't have a negative effect on heart disease risk. Low-carb diets also increase the amount of HDL in the blood.

Triglycerides are another type of fat or lipid that circulates in the blood. The main function of triglycerides is to provide you with energy in between meals, but when you have too many triglycerides in your blood, it becomes a problem. Like small-particle LDL, a high level of triglycerides is a major risk factor for heart disease. It was previously believed that dietary fat and cholesterol were the main causes of high triglyceride levels, but studies now show that it's carbohydrates, specifically fructose, and excess calories that increase triglyceride levels. Cutting carbohydrates and replacing them with fat and protein can significantly reduce triglyceride levels.

As if that wasn't enough motivation, low-carb diets have also been shown to reduce high blood pressure, a condition that contributes to heart disease, kidney disease, and decreased brain function and affects approximately one in three American adults.

Metabolic Syndrome

Metabolic syndrome is a diagnosis given when a person has at least three of the aforementioned conditions—high blood pressure, high blood sugar, high levels of visceral fat, and abnormal cholesterol and triglyceride levels—at once. These conditions are dangerous on their own, but when combined, they become an even more destructive force. Low-carb diets have been shown to dramatically improve every single marker associated with metabolic syndrome, whereas low-fat diets make the condition worse.

Better Brain Function

Although the research isn't as extensive as the research for weight loss, blood sugar, and heart health, low-carb diets have also shown promise for improving brain health and function. In one study, older adults who were considered at risk for developing Alzheimer's disease showed improvement in memory after following a low-carb diet for six weeks. Many researchers believe that Alzheimer's disease develops because the brain becomes insulin resistant and unable to use glucose properly, which leads to inflammation and the resulting memory loss and decreased brain function associated with the condition.

CHAPTER 2

Meal Prep 101

In a perfect world, you would be able to cook all your meals fresh at home and sit down to eat them at your leisure, but in today's modern society, that's not the case. Most people eat their meals in a variety of places—at home, at work, and even in the car. There are restaurants everywhere and lots of options for takeout, but unfortunately, most of these options don't fall in line with a healthy eating plan, let alone a low-carb diet. Because of this, preparing healthy meals in advance—lovingly referred to as meal prepping—is absolutely essential to meeting your goals.

The Science of Meal Prepping

Before jumping into the *how* of meal prepping, it's helpful to discuss the *why*. Is there actually a proven benefit to meal prepping? The answer is yes. There are several benefits. Research has found that people who meal prep tend to consume a greater variety of food and have a significantly greater intake of vegetables, salads, and fruits when compared with those who don't meal prep.

In addition, those who spend at least one hour per day (at least seven hours per week) preparing food in advance spend significantly less money on food than those who spend less than an hour each day planning their meals.

Other research found that when you meal prep, you're far more likely to stick to your nutritional guidelines. This is especially helpful when following a low-carb diet because there are no surprises. When you know exactly what's in your meals, you know exactly how many carbohydrates you're eating.

Aside from the scientific research, there's lots of anecdotal evidence on the benefits of meal prepping. Meal prepping equates to less stress around food, since you always know what you're eating and when. Meal prepping also ultimately saves time. You may have to spend a few hours a week preparing your meals for the upcoming days, but you don't have to cook and wash dishes every night after a long day. The trade-off is worth it.

Getting Organized

When it comes to meal prepping, organization is the key to your success. It may seem like a lot of work in the beginning, but the time you take to get yourself organized is time well spent, so don't skip these steps. It's common to prepare meals for three to four days or even the entire week. The number of meals you prepare and the number of days/hours you spend cooking is entirely up to you. No matter what plan you choose, organization is key.

Designing Your Plan

One of the most effective things you can do to get organized is to design your meal plan. You can start on a week-to-week basis, or you can design a schedule for the entire month. Either way, you want to write down exactly what you'll be having for every meal and every snack. You can keep it basic with a notebook and a pen or utilize online meal planners and trackers. There are many free options available. If you're just starting out, it may take a little while to find the system that works best for you, but the more you do this, the easier it will become.

Your schedule may vary, but it's common to set aside an hour or so on a Sunday to sit down, write out your meals, collect the recipes you'll be using, and get your grocery list together. When you start meal planning, it's tempting to go a little overboard looking for fancy recipes or trying to incorporate a lot of variety, but the best thing you can do, at least in the beginning, is keep it simple. Most of the recipes in this book make six servings with easy-to-find ingredients, so if you're meal prepping for one, it only takes a handful of recipes to get you through the bulk of the week.

Writing Your Grocery List

Before writing your grocery list, check your pantry and your refrigerator to see what you have on hand. Make a note of what you already have so you don't pick up extra. (One of the goals is to eliminate waste!) If you prefer, you can even take stock of your refrigerator and pantry before writing your meal plan for the week so you can choose recipes that use up most of the items that you already have on hand.

When you write your grocery list, organize the items on your list by where they are found in the grocery store. That way, you don't have to spend time backtracking while you're shopping or constantly rereading your list to make sure you have everything. Put all produce items together, all canned items together, all meats together, and so on. If there any specialty items that you need to purchase at separate stores or online, put those items on a separate list and categorize them by store/website.

Ordering in Bulk

When you meal prep, you often use some of the same basic ingredients—like chicken breasts, olive oil, almond flour, and coconut milk, for example—repeatedly. You can save yourself time and even money by purchasing these items in larger quantities and stocking up your freezer and pantry. If you don't have one already, purchasing a membership to a wholesale club is a great way to save money and to find these staples in bulk all in one place. Most wholesale clubs are catching on to the growing interest in clean and healthy eating and offering plenty of options for consumers.

ESSENTIAL

Often, stores like T.J. Maxx, Marshalls, and HomeGoods have a food section where you can find specialty food items like coconut oil, coconut flour, avocado oil, nuts, and nut butters for a great price. These stores are constantly changing their inventory, so it's worth a peek to see what they have on a regular basis and stock up on any items that you need or want to try.

Like wholesale clubs, several different websites offer memberships that allow you to purchase healthy food items at a discount. Other websites provide items already discounted and offer periodic discount codes that deepen your savings. Bookmark your favorite websites and check them regularly for sales. When an item that you use regularly goes on sale, purchase a few extra and keep them on hand for when you need them.

Frozen Vegetables

Frozen vegetables are often cheaper than fresh produce, and you can store them longer. As an added bonus, frozen vegetables are often more nutritious because they were picked at peak freshness and frozen immediately, which preserves their nutrients. On the other hand, fresh produce begins losing nutrients as soon as it's picked, and if you purchase it in your local grocery store, sometimes it's been weeks since its picking date. Watch out for sales on frozen vegetables and stock up your freezer when you can.

Storing Your Meals

When meal prepping, proper storage is vital to making sure your food stays fresh and tasty. Proper storage is also helpful if you have to take your meals with you on the go. Spending a little extra time dividing your meals into portions before storing them will save you lots of time when you're ready to eat. After cooking your meals and sides, divide them into six equal portions and put each completed meal in an airtight container. You can store your protein with your side right in the same container. Many of these recipes are designed so that you can pick and choose which items you want to put together. Others are a complete meal on their own.

Once meals are assembled, use a piece of tape to label each meal—Monday breakfast, Monday lunch, Monday dinner, and so on. Many of the meals can also be frozen for later. In addition to taking the time to label food properly, it's important to have the right storage containers. Many companies make airtight stainless steel and glass containers so you can store your food without exposure to plastic. If you choose plastic containers, look for some that are BPA-free and have lids that securely lock in place to keep your food fresh and prevent spills when you're on the go.

Reheating Stored Food

The best way to reheat your stored food to retain moisture and flavor is to warm it through slowly. The easiest way to do this is in a medium skillet on the stovetop or in the oven. If using a skillet, add a little olive oil or ghee to the pan and heat on low until food reaches your desired temperature. If using the oven, reheat with the temperature around 250°F and keep a watchful eye on your meal. If you have a toaster oven, you can use that instead of a conventional oven.

Microwaves are quick and easy, but in some cases, you'll be sacrificing flavor and texture for convenience. If a microwave is your only option, reheat in thirty-second intervals, making sure to stir your food and check the temperature as you go because microwaves cook—and can overcook—food quickly.

A Note on Freezer Meals

There are twenty recipes in this book designated as freezer meals. Each recipe provides instructions for how to properly store the meal, but most of these recipes are designed to prepare in advance, freeze, and then cook at a later time. When storing these freezer meals, it's a good idea to affix a label to the bag or container that has the cooking or reheating instructions written on it. That way, when it comes time to cook the meal, you won't have to go back to the recipe to figure out what to do; you'll have the instructions right there.

If you make it a point to include preparation for at least one freezer meal during each week of your meal prep, you'll be able to fully stock your freezer with months' worth of meals that are ready to thaw and cook. Freezer meals come in really handy if you're a day behind in planning or cooking or on those days when you just don't feel like it.

The Importance of Food Quality

The National Academy of Sciences reports that 90 percent of chemicals applied to foods have never been tested for food safety. When there is no information available on how something will affect you long term, it's best to go by what healthcare professionals call "the precautionary principle"—in other words, when it doubt, leave it out. When following a low-carb diet—or any diet for that matter—it's best to choose organic foods that are free of pesticides and as close to their natural state as possible.

According to a report done by the Environmental Protection Agency, most of the pesticides that humans consume—around 90 percent—come from meat, poultry, fish, eggs, and dairy products. Because low-carb diets tend to contain a decent amount of meat and dairy (if you can tolerate it), it is especially important to choose foods of a higher quality. Look for beef and pork that are organic and grass-fed. Choose dairy products that come from cows that are grass-fed. Purchase chicken and eggs that are organic and pasture-raised. If you have a farm nearby, develop a relationship with your local farmer. Get to know the farm's practices for raising and butchering its animals and support it whenever possible.

ALERT

Animal products contain more pesticides because they're typically higher on the food chain. Animals that consume plants and grains absorb all the toxins and pesticides that have been put on the plants. Animals that eat other animals, such as large fish that eat smaller fish, absorb the toxins from the smaller fish and everything that the smaller fish have eaten.

When choosing vegetables, buy organic whenever possible. If purchasing all organic isn't in your budget, consider what the Environmental Working Group calls "the Dirty Dozen Plus." The "Dirty Dozen Plus" includes:

- Strawberries
- Spinach
- Nectarines
- Apples
- Peaches
- Pears
- Cherries
- Grapes
- Celery
- Tomatoes
- Bell peppers
- Potatoes
- Hot peppers

These are the fruits and vegetables most likely to contain high levels of pesticides. Prioritize purchasing organic versions of these whenever possible.

Once you get into the groove of meal prepping for a low-carb diet, you're going to wonder why you didn't start sooner. You'll experience lower levels of stress, you'll save money, you'll consume a wider variety of nutrients, and you'll be lowering your risk of diabetes and heart disease. That's a combination that can't be beat.

CHAPTER 3

Breakfast

Coconut Chia Pudding

The longer this chia pudding sits in the refrigerator, the thicker it gets. If you prefer it a little thinner, you can stir in a touch more coconut milk right before you eat it. You can store this chia pudding in the refrigerator up to 4 days.

INGREDIENTS | SERVES 6

1½ cups chia seeds

6 cups full-fat coconut milk

3 teaspoons ground cinnamon

18 drops liquid stevia

Choosing a Stevia

Stevia can be a healthy low-carb sweetener choice, but not all stevia is created equally. Look for stevia that is "whole leaf," which means it was minimally processed and doesn't contain maltodextrin or dextrose.

1. Combine ¼ cup chia seeds, 1 cup coconut milk, ½ teaspoon cinnamon, and 3 drops liquid stevia in six separate glass jars with lids. Mason jars work really well.

2. Stir until ingredients are evenly combined. Cover each jar with a lid and let sit 6 hours or overnight.

3. Serve cold.

PER SERVING   Calories: 587 | Fat: 59 g | Protein: 12 g | Sodium: 29 mg | Fiber: 9 g | Carbohydrates: 17 g | Sugar: 0 g

Cauliflower Hash Browns

These cauliflower hash browns are delicious hot or cold. You can heat them up quickly in a little bit of oil right before you eat them, or you can eat them right out of the refrigerator. These hash browns will last up to 1 week in the refrigerator.

INGREDIENTS | SERVES 6

1½ pounds cauliflower florets, shredded

4 large eggs

½ medium yellow onion, peeled and finely minced

¼ teaspoon freshly ground black pepper

Ghee, for frying

1. Combine all ingredients except ghee in a medium bowl and allow to sit 10 minutes.

2. Heat up ghee in a large skillet over medium heat. Scoop cauliflower mixture into pan and flatten into circles about 3"–4" in diameter.

3. Cook 4–5 minutes on each side or until lightly browned.

4. Divide evenly into six airtight containers and store in the refrigerator until ready to eat.

PER SERVING   Calories: 116 | Fat: 7 g | Protein: 7 g | Sodium: 81 mg | Fiber: 3 g | Carbohydrates: 7 g | Sugar: 2.5 g

Cauliflower Skillet Casserole

Cauliflower doesn't make its way onto breakfast plates a lot, but the vegetable is so versatile that it goes with practically anything. Although this is designed as a breakfast meal, it's perfect for any meal of the day. This dish will last up to 1 week in the refrigerator.

INGREDIENTS | SERVES 6

1 tablespoon olive oil
1 small yellow onion, peeled and diced
12 ounces ground no-sugar-added chicken sausage
2 cups chopped cauliflower florets
½ teaspoon salt
¼ teaspoon freshly ground black pepper
¼ teaspoon ground sage
12 large eggs
½ cup coconut milk
½ cup shredded Cheddar cheese
3 tablespoons chopped green onions

1. Preheat oven to 350°F.

2. Heat olive oil in a large skillet over medium heat. Add onions and sausage and cook until sausage is no longer pink, about 6 minutes. Add cauliflower and continue cooking until cauliflower is softened, about 5 minutes.

3. Season with salt, pepper, and sage and stir until combined.

4. In a separate medium bowl, whisk together eggs and coconut milk. Pour eggs into skillet over sausage and cauliflower mixture. Stir gently to combine.

5. Sprinkle cheese on top of mixture and transfer skillet to oven.

6. Bake in oven 45 minutes or until eggs are set.

7. Top with green onions and allow to cool. Cut into six pieces and store in separate airtight containers in the refrigerator until ready to eat, up to 1 week.

PER SERVING   Calories: 383 | Fat: 29 g | Protein: 26 g | Sodium: 466 mg | Fiber: 1 g | Carbohydrates: 4 g | Sugar: 1.5 g

Kale and Sausage Egg Cups

Egg cups are one of the best meal prep breakfasts because they're easy to make in bulk, and you can incorporate tons of your favorite vegetables. They also keep well in the refrigerator up to 1 week and can even be frozen.

INGREDIENTS | SERVES 6 (MAKES 12 EGG CUPS)

1 tablespoon olive oil

1 clove garlic, minced

½ medium white onion, peeled and minced

¼ pound hot no-sugar-added Italian sausage

4 cups chopped kale

12 large eggs

½ teaspoon salt

¼ teaspoon freshly ground black pepper

4 ounces crumbled feta cheese

Freezing Egg Cups

If you want to freeze your egg cups so they last even longer, all you have to do is allow them to cool completely, wrap each individual egg cup in plastic wrap, and then place each wrapped egg cup in a freezer bag or airtight container. Frozen egg cups are good up to 2 months.

1. Preheat oven to 350°F.

2. Heat olive oil in a medium skillet over medium heat. Add garlic and onion and cook until translucent, about 3 minutes. Add sausage and cook until no longer pink, about 7 minutes.

3. Add kale to skillet and cook until wilted, about 5 minutes.

4. Whisk eggs with salt and pepper in a medium bowl. Add sausage mixture to eggs and stir gently until combined.

5. Spray muffin tin with nonstick baking spray and transfer egg mixture into each well evenly. Sprinkle feta cheese on top.

6. Bake 25 minutes or until eggs are set and toothpick inserted in center comes out clean.

7. Transfer two egg cups into each of six airtight containers or snack bags and store in the refrigerator until ready to eat.

PER SERVING Calories: 275 | Fat: 20 g | Protein: 19 g | Sodium: 649 mg | Fiber: 1 g | Carbohydrates: 3 g | Sugar: 2 g

Cinnamon Swirl Muffins

Muffins are great to have on hand when meal prepping because they're easy to eat on the go. Don't let the cauliflower in this recipe scare you off; you can't even taste it! These muffins will last 1 week at room temperature.

INGREDIENTS | SERVES 6 (MAKES 12 MUFFINS)

1 cup cooked cauliflower, cooled

¾ cup vanilla protein powder

½ cup no-sugar-added powdered peanut butter

3 large eggs

1 tablespoon coconut oil

½ teaspoon plus 2 drops liquid stevia, divided

1 teaspoon baking powder

2 tablespoons ghee

1 tablespoon cinnamon

1. Preheat oven to 350°F.

2. Combine all ingredients except 2 drops stevia, ghee, and cinnamon in a blender and blend until batter is smooth.

3. Spray a 12-cup muffin tin with nonstick baking spray. Fill each well evenly with muffin mixture.

4. In a small saucepan, melt ghee over medium heat. Add 2 drops liquid stevia and cinnamon and stir until combined.

5. Top each muffin with ½ teaspoon of cinnamon mixture and swirl with a toothpick.

6. Bake 10 minutes or until toothpick inserted in center comes out clean.

7. Transfer two muffins into each of six airtight containers or snack bags and store at room temperature until ready to eat.

PER SERVING Calories: 229 | Fat: 20 g | Protein: 8 g | Sodium: 211 mg | Fiber: 2 g | Carbohydrates: 7 g | Sugar: 3 g

Choosing a Protein Powder

A lot of protein powders are loaded with sweeteners and aren't compatible with a low-carb diet. Others are low in carbohydrates but still contain artificial sweeteners that aren't good for you. Make sure to check your labels when choosing a vanilla protein powder and choose one that contains only natural, carbohydrate-free sweeteners like stevia. If you're okay with dairy, Primal Kitchen makes a great protein powder called Primal Fuel. If you'd rather avoid dairy, try the Designs for Health PurePaleo line.

Bacon Spinach Egg Cups

This recipe can also be easily adapted into a frittata by pouring the eggs directly into an 8" × 8" baking dish and baking about 30 minutes or until eggs are set. Once cooled, all you have to do is cut into six equal-sized portions, and you're set with a week's worth of breakfast.

INGREDIENTS | SERVES 6 (MAKES 12 EGG CUPS)

4 slices no-sugar-added bacon, diced
1 cup chopped spinach
4 whole white mushrooms, chopped
2 tablespoons minced onion
2 tablespoons minced green bell pepper
12 large eggs
½ teaspoon salt
¼ teaspoon freshly ground black pepper
⅛ teaspoon onion powder
⅛ teaspoon garlic powder

Find a Good Bacon

All bacon is not created equally. The bacon that's easily accessible in most stores may be filled with sugar and other undesirable ingredients like nitrates, which, when exposed to high heat, have been linked to cancer. When looking for a nitrate-free, no-sugar-added bacon, it's best to start at your local farm or butcher. You may be able to request a special batch. If you're unsuccessful there, you can purchase some online from Pederson's Natural Farms.

1. Preheat oven to 350°F.

2. Cook bacon in a medium skillet over medium heat. Once bacon is crisp, remove from skillet and set aside.

3. Add spinach, mushrooms, onion, and bell pepper to pan with bacon grease and cook over medium heat until spinach is wilted and bell peppers are soft, about 4 minutes. Remove from heat.

4. Whisk together eggs, salt, pepper, onion powder, and garlic powder in a medium bowl. Chop bacon and add to egg mixture. Fold in spinach mixture.

5. Spray a 12-cup muffin tin with nonstick baking spray and transfer egg mixture to wells evenly.

6. Bake 20 minutes or until eggs are set and toothpick inserted in center comes out clean.

7. Transfer two egg cups into each of six airtight containers or snack bags and store in the refrigerator until ready to eat, up to 1 week.

PER SERVING   Calories: 225 | Fat: 17 g | Protein: 15 g | Sodium: 464 mg | Fiber: 0.5 g | Carbohydrates: 2 g | Sugar: 1 g

Bacon Pancakes

These aren't your typical sweet pancakes. The bacon and chive combo gives them a savory flavor that's out of this world. When dividing these pancakes up during your meal prep, you can also top them with a dollop or two of Coconut Sour Cream (Chapter 9). These pancakes will last 1 week in the refrigerator.

INGREDIENTS | SERVES 6 (3 PANCAKES PER SERVING)

6 slices no-sugar-added bacon
9 large egg whites
¾ cup coconut flour
3 tablespoons grass-fed gelatin
6 tablespoons ghee, melted
3 tablespoons dried chives
1½ cups coconut milk

Benefits of Gelatin

Gelatin is a unique protein that provides important amino acids that help improve gut health, protect joints, improve quality of sleep, boost mood, and contribute to healthy skin. It's important to choose a high-quality, grass-fed gelatin, like the one from Vital Proteins.

1. Cook bacon in a medium skillet over medium-high heat. Remove bacon from pan and set aside to cool. Reserve bacon grease.

2. Put egg whites in a medium bowl and beat with an electric mixer until soft peaks form.

3. Roughly chop cooled bacon.

4. In a separate medium bowl, combine coconut flour, gelatin, ghee, chives, and bacon. Add coconut milk and mix well. Fold egg whites into mixture.

5. Reheat reserved bacon grease over medium heat. Drop 2 tablespoons of pancake batter into heated skillet and form into a pancake. Cook 2–3 minutes on each side or until golden brown.

6. Transfer three pancakes into each of six airtight containers or snack bags and store in the refrigerator until ready to eat.

PER SERVING   Calories: 392 | Fat: 37 g | Protein: 12 g | Sodium: 275 mg | Fiber: 9 g | Carbohydrates: 12 g | Sugar: 0.5 g

Flourless Zucchini Muffins

Don't let the zucchini in these muffins scare you away. Zucchini is extremely versatile and can be easily hidden in recipes for an extra nutrient boost. It also helps keep this recipe moist so it has a longer shelf life, which is perfect for meal prep. The muffins will last up to 1 week in the refrigerator.

INGREDIENTS | SERVES 6

½ cup no-sugar-added creamy almond butter

1 medium very ripe banana

¼ cup unsweetened cocoa powder

¼ teaspoon liquid stevia

2 tablespoons ground flaxseed

1 teaspoon vanilla extract

½ teaspoon baking soda

1 cup shredded zucchini, strained

Straining Your Zucchini

Straining your zucchini is important, so don't skip that step! You can easily strain zucchini by placing shreds in a cheesecloth or nut bag and squeezing until all the excess water is removed. If you don't have a cheesecloth or a nut bag, use a paper towel and squeeze out as much as you can.

1. Preheat oven to 375°F.

2. Combine all ingredients except zucchini in a blender and blend until batter is completely smooth.

3. Transfer to a medium bowl and stir in shredded zucchini.

4. Spray a 12-cup muffin tin with nonstick cooking spray and fill wells ¾ of the way full.

5. Bake 30 minutes or until toothpick inserted in center comes out clean.

6. Transfer two muffins into each of six airtight containers or snack bags and store in the refrigerator until ready to eat.

PER SERVING   Calories: 170 | Fat: 12 g | Protein: 7 g | Sodium: 198 mg | Fiber: 4 g | Carbohydrates: 12 g | Sugar: 5 g

Coconut Cream with Low-Carb Granola

If you like crispy granola, it's best to follow this recipe exactly as written. If you like your granola softened, you can store the granola right on top of the coconut cream in your meal prep containers. This dish will last up to 1 week in the refrigerator.

INGREDIENTS | SERVES 6

4 ounces chopped almonds

⅓ cup unsweetened shredded coconut

½ cup raw sunflower seeds

2 tablespoons pumpkin seeds

⅓ cup whole flaxseeds

½ tablespoon ground cinnamon

½ tablespoon pumpkin pie spice

1 teaspoon vanilla extract

4 tablespoons almond flour

½ cup water

2 tablespoons coconut oil

3 cups coconut cream

What Is Coconut Cream?

There are two distinct layers in a can of full-fat coconut milk—a solid layer on top and a liquid layer on the bottom. In recipes that call for coconut cream, use only the solid portion of the can of coconut milk. In recipes that call for coconut milk, blend the solid and liquid layers together before using. Some stores also sell canned coconut cream, but in many cases, these cans contain sweeteners. Check labels thoroughly before using.

1. Preheat oven to 300°F. Line a baking sheet with parchment paper.

2. Mix all ingredients except coconut cream in a large bowl. Spread out on baking sheet.

3. Roast 20 minutes. Remove from oven and stir mixture. Return to oven 20 more minutes. Remove from oven and stir.

4. Return baking sheet to oven and turn off heat. Let granola cool in oven while oven is cooling down.

5. Divide coconut cream evenly into six airtight containers. Divide granola equally into six snack bags and place closed snack bags in containers. Store in the refrigerator until ready to eat.

PER SERVING   Calories: 530 | Fat: 50 g | Protein: 12 g | Sodium: 18 mg | Fiber: 7 g | Carbohydrates: 14 g | Sugar: 2 g

Low-Carb Waffles

These waffles can be enjoyed cold, but if you prefer to reheat them, just pop them in the toaster for a few minutes right before eating. They'll last up to 1 week in the refrigerator.

INGREDIENTS | SERVES 6 (1 WAFFLE PER SERVING)

12 large egg whites
6 large eggs
¾ cup coconut flour
¾ cup full-fat coconut milk
3 teaspoons baking powder
½ teaspoon liquid stevia

1. Heat up a waffle iron.

2. Place egg whites in a medium bowl and beat with an electric hand mixer until stiff peaks form.

3. Add remaining ingredients and stir until combined.

4. Spray heated waffle iron with nonstick cooking spray. Pour batter onto waffle iron in ⅛ cup measurements. Cook until browned, about 3 minutes.

5. Transfer one waffle into each of six airtight containers and store in the refrigerator until ready to eat.

PER SERVING Calories: 188 | Fat: 12 g | Protein: 16 g | Sodium: 428 mg | Fiber: 9 g | Carbohydrates: 12 g | Sugar: 0.5 g

N'oatmeal

This N'oatmeal thickens the longer it sits in the refrigerator because the chia seeds gel and expand. If you prefer it a little thinner, just add a little more almond or coconut milk right before you eat it. This dish will last in the refrigerator for up to 1 week.

INGREDIENTS | SERVES 6

¾ cup chia seeds
¾ cup unsweetened shredded coconut
1 cup coconut flakes
½ cup slivered almonds
4 tablespoons powered erythritol
3 teaspoons vanilla extract
1½ cups full-fat coconut milk
3 cups unsweetened almond milk
7 drops liquid stevia

1. Combine chia seeds, shredded coconut, coconut flakes, almonds, and erythritol in a medium bowl and mix thoroughly. Add vanilla extract, coconut milk, almond milk, and stevia and stir until combined.

2. Let sit 15 minutes and then split evenly among six glass jars with lids. Store in the refrigerator until ready to eat.

PER SERVING Calories: 513 | Fat: 50 g | Protein: 9 g | Sodium: 24 mg | Fiber: 7 g | Carbohydrates: 21 g | Sugar: 1.5 g

Egg Frittata

Frittatas are a great way to use up all the fresh vegetables in your refrigerator at the end of your week. This basic recipe is easily adaptable, so feel free to throw in whatever extra low-carb vegetables you have. This frittata will keep in the refrigerator for 1 week.

INGREDIENTS | SERVES 6

12 large eggs
2 tablespoons coconut milk
½ cup chopped seeded tomatoes
¼ cup chopped fresh basil
½ teaspoon salt
¼ teaspoon freshly ground black pepper
3 tablespoons feta cheese

1. Preheat oven to 350°F.

2. Whisk eggs and coconut milk together in a medium bowl. Add tomatoes, basil, salt, and pepper and whisk until combined.

3. Spray a 9" pie plate with nonstick cooking spray. Pour egg mixture into prepared pie plate. Sprinkle with feta cheese.

4. Bake 30 minutes or until toothpick inserted in center comes out clean.

5. Cut into six equal portions and transfer each portion to an airtight container. Store in the refrigerator until ready to eat.

PER SERVING Calories: 25 | Fat: 2 g | Protein: 1 g | Sodium: 238 mg | Fiber: 0.5 g | Carbohydrates: 1 g | Sugar: 0.5 g

Blueberry Muffins

The lemon extract really complements the blueberries in these muffins, but if you don't have any easily accessible, you can use vanilla extract instead and get equally delicious results. These muffins will last 1 week at room temperature.

INGREDIENTS | SERVES 6 (MAKES 12 MUFFINS)

1 cup almond flour

½ cup coconut flour

2 teaspoons baking powder

½ teaspoon salt

4 tablespoons melted ghee

6 large eggs

½ cup almond milk

4 tablespoons powdered erythritol

¼ teaspoon liquid stevia

1 teaspoon lemon extract

¾ cup blueberries

What Is Erythritol?

Erythritol is a sugar substitute that contains no calories and no carbohydrates. It's a common replacement for sugar on low-carb diets because it measures almost cup for cup (you have to use slightly more erythritol to get the same sweetness), and it doesn't have the unpleasant digestive side effects common with other sugar alcohols like xylitol.

1. Combine almond flour, coconut flour, baking powder, and salt in a small bowl. In a separate medium bowl, whisk together melted ghee, eggs, almond milk, erythritol, stevia, and lemon extract.

2. Fold dry ingredients into wet ingredients and mix until just combined. Fold in blueberries.

3. Spray a 12-cup muffin tin with nonstick baking spray. Fill each well ¾ of the way full.

4. Bake 25 minutes or until toothpick inserted in center comes out clean.

5. Place two muffins in each of six airtight containers or snack bags and store at room temperature until ready to eat.

PER SERVING   Calories: 319 | Fat: 28 g | Protein: 12 g | Sodium: 430 mg | Fiber: 8 g | Carbohydrates: 22 g | Sugar: 2 g

Smoked Salmon Deviled Eggs

Avocados start to brown after a day or so in the refrigerator. You can increase the amount of time they stay green by squeezing a little lemon juice on top of the slices right after you cut them. These eggs will keep in the refrigerator up to 1 week.

INGREDIENTS | SERVES 6

12 large hard-boiled eggs

3 teaspoons hot sauce

¾ cup Basic Mayonnaise (Chapter 9)

¼ teaspoon salt

2 tablespoons chopped fresh dill

12 strips smoked salmon

½ medium avocado, cut into 12 slices

1. Carefully cut hard-boiled eggs in half and transfer yolks to a small bowl.

2. Mash yolks with a fork and add hot sauce, mayonnaise, salt, and dill and continue mashing until combined.

3. Scoop yolk mixture back into egg whites. Cut salmon strips in half and top each prepared egg half with a piece of salmon and a slice of avocado.

4. Place four halves in each of six airtight containers and store in the refrigerator until ready to eat.

PER SERVING Calories: 143 | Fat: 9.5 g | Protein: 13 g | Sodium: 301 mg | Fiber: 0 g | Carbohydrates: 1 g | Sugar: 0.5 g

Low-Carb Pancakes

You can double or triple this pancake recipe, store extras in the freezer, and heat them up right when you're ready to eat. All you have to do is take them out of the freezer and put them directly into the toaster. If stored in the refrigerator, pancakes will last up to 6 days.

INGREDIENTS | SERVES 6 (MAKES 12 PANCAKES)

1 cup blanched almond flour

¼ cup coconut flour

2 tablespoons erythritol

1 teaspoon baking powder

6 large eggs

6 tablespoons coconut milk

1 teaspoon vanilla extract

⅛ teaspoon sea salt

2 tablespoons coconut oil

1. Mix all ingredients except coconut oil in a medium bowl.

2. Heat coconut oil in a medium skillet over medium heat. Drop batter into pan to form circles about 5" in diameter. Cook on one side until bubbles start to form, about 3 minutes. Once bubbles form, flip and cook another 2–3 minutes on the other side until lightly browned. Repeat with remaining batter until all pancakes are made.

3. Store pancakes in an airtight container in the refrigerator or freezer and reheat when ready to eat.

PER SERVING Calories: 256 | Fat: 22 g | Protein: 11 g | Sodium: 202 mg | Fiber: 5 g | Carbohydrates: 12 g | Sugar: 1 g

Cowboy Skillet

If you don't have an oven-safe skillet, you can turn this into a cowboy scramble by whisking the eggs together before adding them to the pan and then stirring until the eggs are cooked through. This won't affect storage time of 1 week.

INGREDIENTS | SERVES 6

1 tablespoon olive oil

1 pound no-sugar-added breakfast sausage

1 cup chopped cauliflower florets

¼ cup chopped white mushrooms

6 large eggs

½ teaspoon salt

¼ teaspoon freshly ground black pepper

1 medium avocado, pitted, peeled, and thinly sliced

¼ cup chopped cilantro

3 tablespoons hot sauce

What's in a Name?

Cowboy skillets were originally named for the fact that they're so hearty and calorie rich, they could even fill up the stomach of a cowboy. This skillet has all the delicious flavors of a typical cowboy skillet, but it's lower in both calories and carbohydrates.

1. Preheat oven to 400°F.

2. Heat olive oil in a large oven-safe skillet over medium heat. Add sausage and cook until no longer pink, about 6 minutes. Add cauliflower and mushrooms, cover, and cook until softened, about 4 minutes, stirring occasionally.

3. Remove from heat. Spread mixture evenly in pan and form six wells for eggs. Crack each egg directly into a well. Sprinkle with salt and pepper.

4. Set oven to broil and place skillet on top rack. Cook until eggs set, about 5 minutes.

5. Remove skillet from oven and top with avocado, cilantro, and hot sauce.

6. Cut into six equal portions and transfer each portion to an airtight container. Store in the refrigerator until ready to eat.

PER SERVING Calories: 311 | Fat: 25 g | Protein: 18 g | Sodium: 1,009 mg | Fiber: 1 g | Carbohydrates: 2 g | Sugar: 1 g

Coffee Protein Muffins

The coconut yogurt in these muffins helps keep them moist until you're ready to eat them. They hold up best in the refrigerator for 1 week, but if you prefer them softer, allow each individual portion to come to room temperature before you eat it.

INGREDIENTS | SERVES 6 (MAKES 12 MUFFINS)

1½ cups blanched almond flour

¼ cup plus 2 tablespoons vanilla protein powder

1½ teaspoons baking powder

¼ cup plus 2 tablespoons plain Coconut Yogurt (Chapter 15)

¼ cup plus 2 tablespoons almond or coconut milk

1 large egg

1 large egg white

1½ teaspoons vanilla extract

1½ ounces brewed coffee

7 drops liquid stevia

1. Preheat oven to 350°F.

2. Combine all ingredients in a blender and blend until smooth.

3. Spray a 12-cup muffin tin with nonstick baking spray and fill each well ¾ of the way full.

4. Bake 10–15 minutes or until toothpick inserted in center comes out clean.

5. Allow to cool completely. Transfer two muffins into each of six airtight containers or snack bags and store in the refrigerator until ready to eat.

PER SERVING Calories: 206 | Fat: 18 g | Protein: 8 g | Sodium: 144 mg | Fiber: 3 g | Carbohydrates: 7 g | Sugar: 1 g

Hidden Sugar

Flavored yogurts are a big source of hidden sugar. In fact, some flavored yogurts have as much sugar as a can of soda. Make sure that the yogurt you use in this recipe has no added sugar to stay within your carbohydrate allotment.

Baked Bacon Omelet

Omelets and frittatas are a great opportunity for you to use up your frozen vegetables. If you have frozen spinach, thaw it out and squeeze out excess water before adding it to this recipe. This omelet will keep up to 1 week in the refrigerator.

INGREDIENTS | SERVES 6

½ pound no-sugar-added bacon

2 cups chopped spinach

½ small yellow onion, peeled and chopped

12 large eggs

½ teaspoon salt

¼ teaspoon freshly ground black pepper

3 tablespoons chopped fresh chives

2 tablespoons grated Parmesan cheese

1. Preheat oven to 400°F. Grease an 8" × 8" glass baking dish with nonstick baking spray.

2. Heat a medium skillet over medium heat. Cook bacon until crispy and transfer to paper towel to cool. Return pan to heat. Add spinach and onion to bacon grease and cook until translucent, about 4 minutes. Remove from heat.

3. Chop bacon and toss into spinach mixture. Stir until combined.

4. Whisk eggs with salt and pepper in a large bowl until frothy. Pour eggs into baking dish and evenly spread bacon and spinach mixture on top.

5. Sprinkle chives and Parmesan cheese on top. Cook 20 minutes or until toothpick inserted in center comes out clean.

6. Cut into six equal portions and put each portion in a separate airtight container. Store in the refrigerator until ready to eat.

PER SERVING Calories: 317 | Fat: 25 g | Protein: 19 g | Sodium: 638 mg | Fiber: 0.5 g | Carbohydrates: 2.5 g | Sugar: 1 g

Lemon Poppy Seed Muffins

Poppy seeds are not just for show—they contain essential fatty acids called oleic and linoleic acid that help reduce LDL cholesterol and protect your heart. They're also rich in fiber and B vitamins. Muffins will last up to 1 week at room temperature.

INGREDIENTS | SERVES 6 (MAKES 12 MUFFINS)

4 large eggs, separated
½ cup full-fat coconut milk
6 tablespoons granulated erythritol
2 large Meyer lemons, zested and juiced
2 teaspoons baking powder
3 cups blanched almond flour
2 teaspoons poppy seeds

1. Preheat oven to 350°F.

2. Combine egg yolks, coconut milk, erythritol, lemon zest, and baking powder in a large mixing bowl. Stir in almond flour and lemon juice.

3. In a separate medium bowl, beat egg whites with an electric mixer until soft peaks form. Add 1 tablespoon of beaten egg whites to egg yolk mixture and stir until combined. Fold in remaining egg whites. Fold in poppy seeds.

4. Spray a 12-cup muffin tin with nonstick baking spray and divide mixture evenly among the 12 wells.

5. Bake 15 minutes or until toothpick inserted in center comes out clean.

6. Store two muffins in each of six airtight containers.

PER SERVING Calories: 410 | Fat: 35 g | Protein: 17 g | Sodium: 212 mg | Fiber: 6 g | Carbohydrates: 25 g | Sugar: 2 g

Breakfast Casserole

Breakfast casseroles are a great way to use up leftover groceries in your refrigerator. If you don't have all the ingredients in this casserole, you can swap other low-carbohydrate vegetables to make it your own. This casserole will keep in the refrigerator up to 6 days.

INGREDIENTS | SERVES 6

1 tablespoon olive oil

1 tablespoon minced garlic

½ cup diced yellow onion

¾ cup diced red bell pepper

¾ cup diced green bell pepper

12 ounces ground no-sugar-added breakfast sausage

2 cups baby spinach, chopped

12 large eggs

½ teaspoon salt

¼ teaspoon freshly ground black pepper

½ cup shredded Cheddar cheese

1. Preheat oven to 350°F.

2. Heat olive oil in a medium pan over medium heat. Add garlic and onion and cook until translucent, about 3 minutes. Add peppers and cook until softened, about 5 minutes.

3. Crumble ground sausage into pan and cook until sausage is no longer pink, about 7 minutes. Add spinach and continue cooking until wilted, about 2 minutes.

4. Remove from heat.

5. In a large bowl, whisk eggs with salt and pepper. Add sausage mixture and gently stir until combined.

6. Transfer egg mixture to a 9" × 9" baking dish and top with cheese.

7. Bake 45 minutes or until eggs are cooked all the way through and a knife comes out clean. Cut into six equal portions and transfer each portion into a separate airtight container. Store in the refrigerator until ready to eat.

PER SERVING   Calories: 387 | Fat: 29 g | Protein: 25 g | Sodium: 831 mg | Fiber: 1.5 g | Carbohydrates: 5.5 g | Sugar: 3 g

CHAPTER 4

Poultry

Bacon Turkey Burgers

Once cooked, these turkey burgers will last in the refrigerator up to 6 days. If you want to store the burgers in the freezer, put them in the freezer after you've shaped them into patties, but before cooking. They'll stay frozen up to 6 months.

INGREDIENTS | SERVES 6

½ pound no-sugar-added bacon, cooked and diced

2 pounds ground turkey

1 large zucchini, shredded

½ medium yellow onion, peeled and diced

2 cloves garlic, minced

1 teaspoon salt

½ teaspoon freshly ground black pepper

1 teaspoon onion powder

2 tablespoons olive oil

1. Preheat oven to 350°F.

2. Combine all ingredients except olive oil in a large bowl and mix with your hands until evenly combined. Form into six equal-sized patties.

3. Heat olive oil in medium skillet over medium heat. Cook patties 3 minutes on each side or until browned.

4. Transfer browned patties to a baking sheet lined with parchment paper and bake in oven 15 minutes or until internal temperature reaches 165°F. Transfer each burger to a separate airtight container and store in the refrigerator.

PER SERVING Calories: 432 | Fat: 30 g | Protein: 34 g | Sodium: 726 mg | Fiber: 1 g | Carbohydrates: 4 g | Sugar: 2 g

Make It a Meatloaf

If you want to save some time during your meal prep, you can turn these burgers into a meatloaf. The zucchini works the same as bread crumbs would to keep the meat moist and fluffy. Once everything is mixed, spread in a 9" × 5" loaf pan and bake at 350°F for about 45 minutes or until turkey is cooked through. Once cooled, cut into six equal portions and transfer each portion to an airtight container.

Teriyaki Chicken and Broccoli

The small amount of orange juice in this recipe is just enough to give this dish added flavor but not enough to drastically affect your carbohydrate count. This recipe will keep in the refrigerator up to 6 days.

INGREDIENTS | SERVES 6

¼ cup coconut aminos
2 tablespoons granulated erythritol
2 tablespoons rice vinegar
1 tablespoon sesame oil
1 tablespoon fresh grated ginger
2 cloves garlic, minced
⅛ teaspoon crushed red pepper flakes
½ teaspoon arrowroot powder
2 tablespoons fresh orange juice
2 tablespoons olive oil
1½ pounds boneless, skinless chicken breasts, cubed
1 teaspoon salt
½ teaspoon freshly ground black pepper
½ teaspoon garlic powder
2 cups broccoli florets
2 tablespoons sesame seeds

Teriyaki Marinade

A company called Coconut Secret, which makes one of the most popular coconut aminos, also makes low-carb, gluten-free, no-sugar-added teriyaki sauce, and it's delicious. If you want to save even more time preparing this recipe, you can replace the first step (and all the ingredients it includes) with this teriyaki sauce.

1. Combine coconut aminos, erythritol, rice vinegar, sesame oil, ginger, garlic, red pepper flakes, arrowroot powder, and orange juice in a small saucepan over medium heat. Bring mixture to a boil and stir constantly 2–3 minutes or until sauce starts to thicken. Remove from heat and allow to cool.

2. Heat olive oil in a medium skillet over medium-high heat. Add chicken cubes, salt, pepper, and garlic powder and cook until no longer pink, about 7 minutes.

3. Pour prepared teriyaki sauce over chicken. Allow to come to a slight boil.

4. Add broccoli florets and toss until completely covered. Cover and allow to cook until broccoli softens, about 3 minutes.

5. Divide cooked chicken and broccoli into six equal portions, sprinkle each with sesame seeds, and store each portion in a separate airtight container. Store in the refrigerator until ready to eat.

PER SERVING   Calories: 240 | Fat: 11 g | Protein: 27 g | Sodium: 738 mg | Fiber: 1.5 g | Carbohydrates: 10 g | Sugar: 1.5 g

Mexican Chicken and Cauliflower Rice

You can save time with this recipe by preparing a bunch of Cauliflower "Rice" (Chapter 13) in your pressure cooker beforehand and using that instead of cooking a new batch of cauliflower rice. This recipe will keep in the refrigerator up to 6 days.

INGREDIENTS | SERVES 6

½ cup almond flour

½ teaspoon salt, divided

¼ teaspoon freshly ground black pepper

½ teaspoon cumin

¼ teaspoon paprika

2 large eggs

6 (4-ounce) boneless, skinless chicken breasts

⅓ cup no-sugar-added salsa

⅓ cup shredded pepper jack cheese

1 large head cauliflower, cut into florets

1 tablespoon olive oil

½ small yellow onion, peeled and diced

2 cloves garlic, minced

1 small green bell pepper, seeded and diced

½ cup petite diced tomatoes

1. Preheat oven to 375°F and line a baking sheet with parchment paper.

2. In a small bowl, combine almond flour, ¼ teaspoon salt, pepper, cumin, and paprika.

3. In a separate small bowl, whisk eggs until frothy.

4. Dip each chicken breast in egg and then almond flour mixture, making sure to completely coat. Place coated chicken breasts on lined baking sheet.

5. Bake 10 minutes, flip each breast over, and then bake another 10 minutes. Remove from oven and spread about 1 tablespoon each of salsa and cheese on top of each chicken breast.

6. Return to oven and bake another 5–7 minutes or until cheese is melted and bubbly.

7. While chicken is cooking, use a food processor with a grater attachment to "rice" cauliflower. Be careful not to overprocess cauliflower or it will become mashed.

8. Heat olive oil in a medium skillet over medium heat. Add onion and garlic and cook until translucent, about 3 minutes. Add green peppers and cook until softened, about 3 more minutes. Stir in cauliflower and remaining salt and cook until just softened. You want the texture to remain similar to cooked rice. Add in tomatoes and stir until combined.

9. Divide cooked cauliflower rice into six equal portions and store with cooked chicken breasts.

PER SERVING Calories: 300 | Fat: 14 g | Protein: 33 g | Sodium: 459 mg | Fiber: 4 g | Carbohydrates: 10 g | Sugar: 4 g

Lemon Chicken Spaghetti Squash

If you're planning to make more than one spaghetti squash dish during your meal prep, you can save time by cooking a couple spaghetti squash at once, scooping out the strands, and storing them in the refrigerator until you're ready to use them. As written, this recipe will keep in the refrigerator up to 6 days.

INGREDIENTS | SERVES 6

1 large spaghetti squash, cut in half lengthwise with seeds scooped out

1½ pounds boneless, skinless chicken breasts

2 tablespoons olive oil

¾ teaspoon salt, divided

¼ teaspoon freshly ground black pepper

2 tablespoons ghee

⅓ cup minced white onion

3 cloves garlic, minced

¾ cup chicken stock

¼ teaspoon arrowroot powder

1½ tablespoons fresh lemon juice

¾ cup coconut cream

½ cup shredded part-skim mozzarella cheese

The Scoop on Arrowroot

Arrowroot powder is a white, tasteless powder that comes from various tubers like the arrowroot plant and cassava plant. It has twice the thickening power of wheat flour, but it's lower in carbohydrates and doesn't contain gluten. Sometimes arrowroot powder will be labeled arrowroot flour, but you can use them interchangeably.

1. Preheat oven to 350°F.

2. Place spaghetti squash face down on baking sheet and bake 45–50 minutes or until tender.

3. While squash is in oven, cover chicken breasts in olive oil, ½ teaspoon salt, and pepper. Place in a 9" × 13" baking dish and place in oven with squash to bake 30 minutes or until juices run clear.

4. While chicken and squash bake, melt ghee in a small saucepan over medium heat. When ghee is melted, add onions and garlic and cook until translucent, about 3 minutes.

5. Add chicken stock and arrowroot powder and cook 4–5 minutes, allowing mixture to thicken and reduce. Stir in lemon juice, coconut cream, and remaining salt.

6. Once squash and chicken are cooked, remove from oven and allow to cool slightly. Remove squash in strands from skin using a fork. Cut chicken into 1" cubes. Transfer squash and chicken to a 9" × 13" baking dish.

7. Pour lemon sauce over chicken and squash and toss until evenly coated.

8. Return dish to oven and bake 25 minutes. Remove from oven, sprinkle with cheese, and return to oven to cook 5 more minutes or until cheese is melted and bubbling.

9. Divide into six equal portions and store each portion in a separate airtight container until ready to eat.

PER SERVING   Calories: 369 | Fat: 22 g | Protein: 30 g | Sodium: 464 mg | Fiber: 2 g | Carbohydrates: 11 g | Sugar: 3 g

Cilantro Lime Chicken

Slitting each chicken breast with a knife before adding the marinade and cooking allows the flavors to really soak into the chicken. This dish will last up to 1 week in the refrigerator.

INGREDIENTS | SERVES 6

1½ pounds boneless, skinless chicken breasts
¼ teaspoon salt
⅛ teaspoon freshly ground black pepper
3 tablespoons olive oil, divided
¼ cup fresh lime juice
⅓ cup chopped fresh cilantro
3 cloves garlic, minced

1. Put three thin slices into each chicken breast with a knife, sprinkle salt and pepper evenly over each breast, and set aside.

2. In a small bowl, whisk together 1 tablespoon olive oil, lime juice, and cilantro.

3. Heat remaining olive oil in a medium skillet over medium heat. Add garlic and cook 1 minute. Add chicken and then pour lime juice mixture on top. Allow to cook 6–7 minutes or until chicken starts to brown and is cooked halfway through. Flip once and continue cooking until juices run clear, about 8 more minutes.

4. Remove from heat and transfer chicken and lime juice mixture to a large bowl. Divide into six equal portions and store in separate airtight containers in the refrigerator until ready to eat.

PER SERVING   Calories: 198 | Fat: 9 g | Protein: 25 g | Sodium: 150 mg | Fiber: 0 g | Carbohydrates: 1 g | Sugar: 0 g

Buffalo Chicken "Rice" Bowl

Poultry seasoning is typically a blend of sage, thyme, marjoram, rosemary, nutmeg, and black pepper. If you don't have a store-bought poultry seasoning, you can season the chicken with any combination of these spices instead. This recipe will keep in the refrigerator up to 6 days.

INGREDIENTS | SERVES 6

1½ pounds boneless, skinless chicken breasts

2 teaspoons poultry seasoning

½ teaspoon garlic powder

½ teaspoon onion powder

1 cup hot sauce

3 tablespoons olive oil, divided

1 tablespoon coconut aminos

1 large head cauliflower, cut into florets

½ small yellow onion, peeled and minced

2 cloves garlic, minced

½ teaspoon salt

¼ teaspoon freshly ground black pepper

¼ cup crumbled blue cheese

Check Your Seasonings!

You may think that seasonings only contain a spice, an herb, or a combination of several, but many seasonings contain added sugar, which will affect your carbohydrate count and your health. Read the labels on the back of any store-bought seasonings you use to make sure the ingredients are clean and don't have any hidden carbohydrates.

1. Preheat oven to 400°F.

2. Place chicken breasts in a 9" × 13" baking dish.

3. In a small bowl, combine poultry seasoning, garlic powder, onion powder, hot sauce, 2 tablespoons olive oil, and coconut aminos. Pour mixture over chicken.

4. Bake 30 minutes or until chicken is cooked all the way through. Remove chicken from oven and shred with a fork. Stir shredded chicken to coat evenly with hot sauce mixture.

5. While chicken is cooking, make cauliflower rice by putting cauliflower through a food processor with a grater attachment.

6. Heat remaining olive oil in a medium skillet over medium heat. Add onion and garlic and cook until translucent, about 4 minutes. Add cauliflower, salt, and pepper and continue to cook until cauliflower is just softened, about 4 more minutes. Remove from heat.

7. Divide cauliflower rice and chicken mixture into six equal portions and put each portion into a separate airtight container. Scoop chicken mixture onto cauliflower rice and sprinkle each portion with blue cheese.

PER SERVING   Calories: 252 | Fat: 11 g | Protein: 28 g | Sodium: 559 mg | Fiber: 2.5 g | Carbohydrates: 7 g | Sugar: 2 g

Broccoli Cheddar Spaghetti Squash Casserole

If you're not using homemade Coconut Yogurt (Chapter 15) for this recipe, look for plain, full-fat coconut milk without any added sugar or artificial sweeteners. If you can't find any and you can tolerate the extra dairy, you can use regular plain yogurt. You can store this dish in the refrigerator up to 6 days.

INGREDIENTS | SERVES 6

1 large spaghetti squash, cut in half lengthwise with the seeds scooped out

3 cups broccoli florets

1 tablespoon olive oil

1 teaspoon salt, divided

½ teaspoon freshly ground black pepper, divided

6 ounces plain coconut yogurt

1 cup shredded Cheddar cheese, divided

¼ cup shredded Parmesan cheese

1 large egg, beaten

1 teaspoon garlic powder

½ teaspoon onion powder

1. Preheat oven to 375°F.

2. Place spaghetti squash cut side down on a baking sheet and bake 45 minutes or until tender. Allow to cool slightly and remove squash in strands from skin with a fork. Transfer spaghetti squash to a 9" × 13" baking dish.

3. Place broccoli on baking sheet and toss with olive oil, ½ teaspoon salt, and ¼ teaspoon pepper. Roast in oven 10 minutes, flipping broccoli over halfway through cooking. Remove from oven.

4. In a medium bowl, combine yogurt, ¾ cup Cheddar cheese, Parmesan cheese, egg, garlic powder, and onion powder and stir until incorporated.

5. Add broccoli to yogurt mixture and toss to combine. Pour broccoli mixture on top of spaghetti squash and stir gently until combined. Add remaining Cheddar cheese on top.

6. Bake 40 minutes or until cheese is slightly browned and casserole is bubbling. Allow to cool and then divide into six equal portions. Store each portion in a separate airtight container in the refrigerator until ready to eat.

PER SERVING   Calories: 222 | Fat: 16 g | Protein: 9 g | Sodium: 569 mg | Fiber: 2.5 g | Carbohydrates: 11 g | Sugar: 2.5 g

Zucchini and Chicken Enchilada Bake

You can replace the canned shredded chicken in this recipe with some Easy Shredded Chicken (Chapter 13) that you prepared in your pressure cooker. You can store this prepared recipe in the refrigerator up to 6 days.

INGREDIENTS | SERVES 6

2 teaspoons olive oil

1 small yellow onion, peeled and minced

2 cloves garlic, minced

2 tablespoons chili powder

1 teaspoon cumin

½ teaspoon paprika

1 teaspoon dried oregano

¼ teaspoon salt

¼ teaspoon freshly ground black pepper

1 (15-ounce) can no-sugar-added tomato sauce

2 tablespoons tomato paste

½ cup no-sugar-added chicken broth

1 teaspoon apple cider vinegar

½ teaspoon arrowroot powder

3 large zucchini

2 (12.5-ounce) cans shredded chicken breast

1 small white onion, peeled and diced

1 small red bell pepper, seeded and diced

1½ cups shredded Cheddar cheese

Sans Mandoline?

A mandoline is the best way to get really thin zucchini slices, but if you don't have one, you can use a sharp knife to cut the zucchini lengthwise as thinly as you can. Watch those fingers, though!

1. Preheat oven to 350°F.

2. Heat olive oil in a medium saucepan over medium heat. Add onion and garlic and cook until translucent, about 4 minutes. Add chili powder, cumin, paprika, oregano, salt, pepper, tomato sauce, tomato paste, chicken broth, vinegar, and arrowroot powder and stir to combine. Bring to a boil and then reduce heat to low. Allow to simmer 5–10 minutes, stirring occasionally, until sauce thickens slightly. Set aside.

3. Slice zucchini lengthwise as thin as possible with a mandoline. Set slices onto a plate lined with a paper towel to absorb excess moisture.

4. Spray a 9" × 9" baking dish with nonstick cooking spray and spread 1 cup enchilada sauce evenly on the bottom. Create a single layer of zucchini slices on top of the sauce, then sprinkle half the chicken, half the onion, half the bell pepper, and ½ cup cheese on top of that. Repeat these layers.

5. Pour any remaining enchilada sauce on top and then cover with remaining ½ cup cheese.

6. Cover with foil and bake 30 minutes. Remove foil and continue baking another 15 minutes or until cheese is slightly browned and casserole is bubbling. Allow to cool slightly and then divide into six equal portions. Place each portion in a separate airtight container and store in the refrigerator until ready to eat.

PER SERVING   Calories: 361 | Fat: 17 g | Protein: 38 g | Sodium: 829 mg | Fiber: 5 g | Carbohydrates: 15 g | Sugar: 9 g

Almond-Crusted Chicken

If you're not a fan of almonds or you can't eat them, cashews make a great substitute for the almonds. If you want to forgo nuts completely, you can use shredded coconut for a sweet, nutty flavor. This dish will keep in the refrigerator up to 6 days.

INGREDIENTS | SERVES 6

1 cup raw almonds
1 teaspoon dried rosemary
¼ teaspoon paprika
½ teaspoon salt
¼ teaspoon freshly ground black pepper
2 large eggs
6 (4-ounce) boneless, skinless chicken breasts
2 tablespoons olive oil

Soak Your Almonds

Raw nuts can cause digestive upset in some people. If you're one of those people, you can alleviate this by soaking your almonds prior to using them. Put 1 cup of almonds in a small bowl and cover with warm water. Let them sit overnight, drain, and lay them out to dry until they're crisp. Make sure to use a bowl that's twice the size of your almonds; as they'll expand significantly while soaking.

1. Preheat oven to 350°F.

2. Using a food processor, coarsely chop almonds. Add rosemary, paprika, salt, and pepper to food processor and pulse until combined. Transfer mixture to a medium bowl.

3. Whisk eggs in a small bowl until frothy.

4. Dip each piece of chicken in egg and then into almond mixture, making sure it's fully coated. Transfer chicken to a clean dish.

5. Heat olive oil in a medium skillet over medium heat and brown each piece of chicken, about 3–4 minutes on each side.

6. Transfer chicken to a 9" × 13" baking dish and bake in oven until fully cooked, about 20 minutes.

7. Divide chicken into six equal portions, combine with your favorite side dish, and store each portion in a separate airtight container in the refrigerator until ready to eat.

PER SERVING Calories: 337 | Fat: 20 g | Protein: 32 g | Sodium: 268 mg | Fiber: 3 g | Carbohydrates: 5 g | Sugar: 1 g

Spinach-and-Feta-Stuffed Chicken Breast

If you want the flavor of this meal without the effort of stuffing the chicken breasts, you can cube the chicken, cook it, and then add the stuffing ingredients right into the pan until incorporated. These stuffed chicken breasts will keep in the refrigerator up to 6 days.

INGREDIENTS | SERVES 6

16 ounces chopped frozen spinach, thawed

¾ cup crumbled feta cheese

4 ounces cream cheese

2 cloves garlic, minced

½ teaspoon salt, divided

¼ teaspoon freshly ground black pepper

6 (4-ounce) chicken breasts

2 tablespoons olive oil

1. Preheat oven to 450°F.

2. Combine spinach, feta cheese, cream cheese, garlic, ¼ teaspoon salt, and pepper in a small bowl. Mix until thoroughly combined.

3. Cut pockets into each chicken breast to prepare for stuffing. Divide spinach mixture into six equal parts and use a spoon to stuff into the pocket of each chicken breast. Secure breasts closed with a toothpick.

4. Sprinkle remaining salt over prepared chicken breasts.

5. Heat olive oil in a large oven-safe pan over medium-high heat. Add chicken breasts and cook 5 minutes or until slightly browned with the top side down.

6. Flip chicken breasts over, move pan to oven, and bake 12 minutes or until juices run clear. Transfer six equal portions to each of six separate airtight containers and store in the refrigerator until ready to eat.

PER SERVING Calories: 310 | Fat: 18 g | Protein: 31 g | Sodium: 539 mg | Fiber: 2 g | Carbohydrates: 5 g | Sugar: 2 g

Chicken Parmesan Spaghetti Squash Casserole

Typically, tomato-based dishes like this casserole taste better after they sit for a couple of days. That's because just like when you simmer a tomato sauce on the stove, the flavors are given the time to meld together in the refrigerator. Store in the refrigerator up to 6 days.

INGREDIENTS | SERVES 6

2 large eggs

½ cup almond flour

⅛ cup grated Parmesan cheese

1 teaspoon salt, divided

½ teaspoon freshly ground black pepper, divided

½ teaspoon garlic powder

½ teaspoon onion powder

2 teaspoons dried parsley, divided

1½ pounds boneless, skinless chicken breasts, cubed

2 tablespoons olive oil

1 large spaghetti squash, cooked and removed from skin

2 cups no-sugar-added marinara sauce

6 ounces shredded part-skim mozzarella cheese

3 tablespoons chopped fresh basil

Finding a Marinara Sauce

Store-bought marinara sauce often has sugar added to it to cut the acidity and to extend the shelf life. If you're using a marinara sauce from the store, read labels diligently until you find one that's appropriate for a low-carb diet. When you do find one that works, buy a few at a time to have them on hand. Combining a jar of marinara sauce with cooked spaghetti squash makes a filling meal in a pinch.

1. Preheat oven to 350°F.

2. Beat eggs in a small bowl. Set aside.

3. In a medium bowl, combine almond flour, Parmesan cheese, ½ teaspoon salt, ¼ teaspoon pepper, garlic powder, onion powder, and 1 teaspoon parsley.

4. Dip chicken a few pieces at a time into egg and then coat with almond flour mixture. Set aside.

5. Heat olive oil over medium heat in a medium skillet and cook chicken until browned on all sides, about 6–7 minutes. Set aside on a plate lined with a paper towel to absorb excess liquid.

6. Combine cooked spaghetti squash; remaining salt, pepper, and parsley; marinara sauce; and cooked chicken in a 9" × 13" baking dish. Toss to make sure spaghetti squash is evenly coated with sauce.

7. Spread spaghetti squash out evenly in the dish and sprinkle mozzarella cheese on top.

8. Bake 30 minutes or until casserole is bubbling. Remove from oven and sprinkle fresh basil on top.

9. Allow to cool slightly and divide into six equal portions. Place each portion in a separate airtight container and store in the refrigerator until ready to eat.

PER SERVING   Calories: 387 | Fat: 23 g | Protein: 37 g | Sodium: 638 mg | Fiber: 2 g | Carbohydrates: 5 g | Sugar: 2 g

Buffalo Chicken Meatballs

These meatballs freeze really well. Once cooked, allow to cool and then transfer meatballs to an airtight container before freezing. If freezing, they'll last in the freezer up to 6 months. If cooked and refrigerated, they'll keep 6 days.

INGREDIENTS | SERVES 6 (MAKES 12 MEATBALLS)

1½ pounds ground chicken

¼ cup almond flour

1 large egg

3 tablespoons minced celery

2 tablespoons crumbled blue cheese

½ teaspoon freshly ground black pepper

⅛ teaspoon garlic powder

6 tablespoons ghee

½ cup plus 2 tablespoons hot sauce

½ teaspoon arrowroot powder

1. Preheat oven to 350°F.

2. Combine all ingredients except ghee, hot sauce, and arrowroot powder in a medium bowl. Mix with your hands until incorporated.

3. Form mixture into 2" balls and place on a baking sheet lined with parchment paper. Bake 12 minutes.

4. While meatballs are baking, combine ghee, hot sauce, and arrowroot powder in a small saucepan over medium heat. Stir constantly while cooking 3 minutes or until sauce thickens slightly. Remove from heat.

5. After meatballs have cooked 12 minutes, remove from oven. Gently toss each ball in prepared buffalo sauce and return to baking sheet. Return to oven and cook another 10–12 minutes or until meatballs reach an internal temperature of 165°F.

6. Put two meatballs in each of six separate airtight containers. Store in the refrigerator until ready to eat.

PER SERVING Calories: 412 | Fat: 35 g | Protein: 21 g | Sodium: 238 mg | Fiber: 1 g | Carbohydrates: 2 g | Sugar: 0.5 g

Chicken Alfredo Spaghetti Squash

This recipe is extremely filling, and it's delicious hot or cold, so it's perfect for meal prep when you have to eat a meal on the go! This Chicken Alfredo Spaghetti Squash will keep in the refrigerator up to 6 days.

INGREDIENTS | SERVES 6

1 large spaghetti squash, cut in half lengthwise

1 tablespoon olive oil

6 tablespoons ghee

2 cloves garlic, minced

3 teaspoons ground sage

5 tablespoons coconut flour

1 teaspoon arrowroot powder

3 cups no-sugar-added chicken broth

1½ cups coconut cream

12 ounces cream cheese

1½ cups shredded Parmesan cheese

1½ cups cooked and shredded chicken

½ teaspoon salt

¼ teaspoon freshly ground black pepper

1 tablespoon chopped fresh parsley

Benefits of Parsley

Parsley is known for being a garnish, but the little green plant is power-packed with nutrition. Just 1 cup of chopped parsley provides over 1,000 percent of your daily needs for vitamin K, which keeps your blood and bones healthy.

1. Preheat oven to 400°F.

2. Drizzle spaghetti squash with olive oil and put cut side down on a baking sheet. Roast 45 minutes or until tender.

3. While squash is cooking, heat ghee in a medium skillet over medium heat. Add garlic and sage and cook until fragrant, about 2 minutes. Stir in coconut flour and arrowroot powder and keep stirring until combined with ghee.

4. Whisk in chicken broth and coconut cream. Stir in cream cheese and Parmesan cheese until smooth. Turn heat to low.

5. Scrape spaghetti squash from skin. Stir spaghetti squash, chicken, salt, pepper, and parsley into cheese mixture. Divide into six equal portions and store each portion in a separate airtight container in the refrigerator.

PER SERVING   Calories: 526 | Fat: 50 g | Protein: 16 g | Sodium: 471 mg | Fiber: 4 g | Carbohydrates: 9 g | Sugar: 2 g

Creamy Chicken Bacon Ranch Casserole

If you like a smoked flavor, you can replace the regular ranch dressing in this recipe with the Bacon Chipotle Ranch Dressing (Chapter 9). Serve on top of a bed of spaghetti squash and you've got a complete meal. This dish will last up to 1 week in the refrigerator.

INGREDIENTS | SERVES 6

1½ pounds chicken breast, cooked and cubed

4 slices no-sugar-added bacon, cooked and roughly chopped

3 cups broccoli florets, steamed and roughly chopped

1 clove garlic, minced

½ cup Ranch Dressing (Chapter 9)

1 cup shredded Cheddar cheese, divided

1. Preheat oven to 375°F.

2. Combine chicken, bacon, broccoli, garlic, ranch dressing, and ½ cup cheese in a 9" × 13" casserole dish. Sprinkle remaining cheese on top.

3. Bake 20–25 minutes or until hot and bubbly.

4. Divide into six equal portions and store each portion in an airtight container in the refrigerator.

PER SERVING Calories: 312 | Fat: 19 g | Protein: 29 g | Sodium: 360 mg | Fiber: 1 g | Carbohydrates: 4 g | Sugar: 2 g

Garlic Chicken

Chicken thighs are not as popular as chicken breasts, so they're often cheaper and go on sale a lot more frequently. You can use chicken thighs in any recipe that calls for breasts if you prefer them. This Garlic Chicken will keep in the refrigerator up to 6 days.

INGREDIENTS | SERVES 6

½ cup ghee

3 tablespoons minced garlic

3 tablespoons coconut aminos

¼ teaspoon arrowroot powder

½ teaspoon freshly ground black pepper

1 tablespoon dried parsley

6 (4-ounce) boneless chicken thighs with skin on

1. Preheat oven to 375°F.

2. Add all ingredients except chicken to a small saucepan. Cook over medium heat stirring constantly until ghee is melted and sauce starts to thicken, about 4 minutes.

3. Coat chicken in garlic mixture and arrange on a baking sheet lined with parchment paper.

4. Bake 45 minutes, turning chicken over and using extra ghee mixture to baste every 15 minutes. Place one chicken thigh into each of six separate airtight containers. Store in the refrigerator until ready to eat.

PER SERVING Calories: 294 | Fat: 20 g | Protein: 25 g | Sodium: 327 mg | Fiber: 0 g | Carbohydrates: 2 g | Sugar: 0 g

Creamy Mustard Chicken

Pair this chicken with Cauliflower Mash (Chapter 10) and you'll have a filling meal that you won't believe is low-carb. You can store this recipe in the refrigerator up to 6 days.

INGREDIENTS | SERVES 6

6 (4-ounce) boneless, skinless chicken breasts

½ teaspoon salt

¼ teaspoon freshly ground black pepper

2 tablespoons olive oil

1 medium yellow onion, peeled and diced

2 cloves garlic, minced

3 cups no-sugar-added chicken broth

¼ cup yellow mustard

¼ teaspoon arrowroot powder

2 tablespoons coconut cream

1 tablespoon ghee

What Is Ghee?

Ghee, which is commonly used in Middle Eastern cuisine, is clarified butter from which the milk solids have been removed. As a result, ghee is free of lactose and has a much higher smoke point, so it can be used in high-temperature cooking. If you tolerate dairy and lactose well, you can substitute butter for ghee in any recipe.

1. Season chicken with salt and pepper. Heat olive oil in a medium skillet over medium heat. Add chicken to skillet and cook 7–8 minutes on each side or until chicken reaches an internal temperature of 165°F.

2. Remove chicken from pan and place on a cutting board to rest.

3. Add onions to oil in pan and cook until translucent, about 4 minutes, scraping pan as you stir. Add garlic and cook another minute. Pour in chicken broth, turn heat to high, and add mustard and arrowroot powder. Cook until reduced by half and slightly thickened, about 5 minutes.

4. Reduce heat to low and add coconut cream and ghee, stirring to combine. Return chicken to pan and coat with mustard sauce.

5. Remove from heat and allow to cool before storing in six airtight containers.

PER SERVING Calories: 218 | Fat: 11 g | Protein: 24 g | Sodium: 392 mg | Fiber: 1 g | Carbohydrates: 3 g | Sugar: 1 g

Chicken Divan

Chicken Divan, which was named after the Divan Parisienne Restaurant, was originally created in New York City. This casserole is a re-creation of that meal but redesigned for meal prep so you can store it in the refrigerator for 1 week.

INGREDIENTS | SERVES 6

1½ pounds boneless, skinless chicken breasts

¼ cup ghee

1 medium yellow onion, peeled and diced

2 cloves garlic, minced

½ teaspoon salt

¼ teaspoon freshly ground black pepper

½ teaspoon curry powder

2 cups riced cauliflower

1 cup no-sugar-added chicken broth

1 cup full-fat coconut milk

1 teaspoon lemon juice

½ cup Basic Mayonnaise (Chapter 9)

2 cups chopped broccoli, steamed

1 cup shredded Cheddar cheese

1 cup shredded mozzarella cheese

¼ cup slivered almonds

Homemade Curry Powder

Curry powder is a combination of spices typically used in Indian cooking. If you don't have store-bought curry powder, you can make your own by combining 4 teaspoons ground coriander, 2 teaspoons turmeric, 1½ teaspoons cumin, ¼ teaspoon black pepper, ¼ teaspoon ground cardamom, ¼ teaspoon ground ginger, ¼ teaspoon ground cinnamon, and ⅛ teaspoon ground cloves. Use what you need and then store the rest in an airtight container in your pantry.

1. Preheat oven to 350°F.

2. Fill a large stockpot halfway with water and bring to a boil over high heat. Add chicken breasts and allow to cook until no longer pink, about 15–20 minutes.

3. While chicken is cooking, heat ghee in a medium skillet over medium heat. Add onions and garlic and cook until they start to soften, about 4 minutes. Add salt, pepper, and curry and stir until onion mixture is coated.

4. Stir in cauliflower and cook until cauliflower starts to soften, about 5 minutes. Stir in chicken broth, cover, and allow to simmer 10 minutes.

5. Add coconut milk and lemon juice and allow to simmer uncovered another 10 minutes, stirring occasionally. Remove from heat and stir in mayonnaise until smooth.

6. Shred your cooked chicken with two forks and mix shredded chicken into riced cauliflower mixture.

7. Line the bottom of an 8" × 8" pan with half the cauliflower mixture, then layer with 1 cup broccoli, ½ cup Cheddar cheese, and ½ cup mozzarella cheese. Put remaining cauliflower mixture on top and then repeat with remaining broccoli and cheese. Sprinkle almond slices on top.

8. Cover with foil and bake 30 minutes. Remove foil and bake another 5–10 minutes or until cheese is slightly browned and bubbling.

9. Allow to cool, then divide into six equal portions. Transfer each portion to an airtight container and store in the refrigerator.

PER SERVING   Calories: 574 | Fat: 44 g | Protein: 35 g | Sodium: 529 mg | Fiber: 3 g | Carbohydrates: 9 g | Sugar: 2.5 g

Baked Chicken with Gravy

Using chicken thighs with the skin on is important in this recipe because the skin creates the extra juices needed to make the gravy. This dish will keep up to 1 week in the refrigerator.

INGREDIENTS | SERVES 6

1½ tablespoons paprika
½ tablespoon chili powder
1 teaspoon onion powder
1 teaspoon garlic powder
1 teaspoon salt
6 medium chicken thighs (about 1½ pounds) with skin on
¼ cup Basic Mayonnaise (Chapter 9)

1. Preheat oven to 375°F.

2. Combine spices in a large mixing bowl. Add chicken thighs to bowl and toss to coat.

3. Transfer chicken to a 9" × 13" baking dish and bake 40 minutes or until chicken is no longer pink.

4. Remove chicken from baking dish and put each thigh into a separate container, reserving juices.

5. Add mayonnaise to baking dish and stir until combined with chicken juices.

6. Pour equal amounts of gravy over each chicken thigh. Cover each container and store in the refrigerator.

PER SERVING   Calories: 309 | Fat: 15 g | Protein: 38 g | Sodium: 644 mg | Fiber: 1 g | Carbohydrates: 2 g | Sugar: 0 g

Turkey and Cauliflower Rice Skillet

If you don't have ground turkey on hand, you can replace it with ground chicken or ground beef for a similar result. This dish will keep up to 1 week in the refrigerator.

INGREDIENTS | SERVES 6

2 tablespoons olive oil

1 small yellow onion, peeled and diced

1 pound white mushrooms, sliced

1 pound ground turkey

1 teaspoon salt

½ teaspoon freshly ground black pepper

3 cups riced cauliflower

2 teaspoons poultry seasoning

1 cup shredded mozzarella cheese

1. Heat olive oil in a medium skillet over medium heat. Add onion and cook until it starts to soften, about 3 minutes. Add mushrooms and continue cooking until softened.

2. Add turkey, salt, and pepper and cook until no longer pink, about 6 minutes. Add cauliflower and poultry seasoning and stir to combine. Continue cooking until softened, about 5 minutes.

3. Sprinkle mozzarella cheese on top and stir until just melted. Remove from heat and allow to cool.

4. Divide into six equal portions and put each portion into an airtight container. Store in the refrigerator.

PER SERVING Calories: 249 | Fat: 15 g | Protein: 21 g | Sodium: 581 mg | Fiber: 3 g | Carbohydrates: 8 g | Sugar: 3 g

Dill Chicken Salad

This dish is easy to whip up and good to have on hand because it's a quick protein source. You can add it to any Mason jar salad in place of the protein or eat it with sliced cucumbers. You can keep this salad in the refrigerator for up to 1 week.

INGREDIENTS | SERVES 6

2 (12.5-ounce) cans cooked chicken breast

½ cup diced celery

2 tablespoons minced white onion

2 large hard-boiled eggs, chopped

¾ cup Basic Mayonnaise (Chapter 9)

½ teaspoon dry mustard powder (or 1 tablespoon Dijon mustard)

2 teaspoons dried dill

½ teaspoon salt

¼ teaspoon freshly ground black pepper

1. Drain cans of chicken and transfer chicken to a medium mixing bowl. Shred with a fork and add remaining ingredients. Mix until combined.

2. Separate into six equal portions and put each portion into an airtight container. Store in the refrigerator.

PER SERVING Calories: 365 | Fat: 26 g | Protein: 28 g | Sodium: 440 mg | Fiber: 0 g | Carbohydrates: 2 g | Sugar: 0 g

CHAPTER 5

Beef

Hamburger Bowls

If you prefer your lettuce crisper, store ¼ cup lettuce in a small snack bag. Make sure the bag is tightly sealed and place the bag in the airtight container with your meat before storing. When you're ready to eat, add lettuce to the cooked beef. These bowls will keep up to 1 week in the refrigerator.

INGREDIENTS | SERVES 6

1 tablespoon olive oil

1½ pounds ground beef

1 teaspoon salt

1 teaspoon freshly ground black pepper

1 teaspoon granulated garlic

1 teaspoon granulated onion

¼ cup Ketchup (Chapter 9)

¼ cup Basic Mayonnaise (Chapter 9)

6 tablespoons chopped pickles

6 tablespoons chopped red onion

1½ cups chopped lettuce

1. Heat olive oil in a medium skillet over medium heat. Add ground beef and spices and cook until meat is no longer pink, about 7 minutes. Remove from heat and stir in ketchup and mayonnaise.

2. Divide cooked meat evenly into six airtight containers. Top each container with 1 tablespoon pickles, 1 tablespoon onions, and ¼ cup chopped lettuce. Cover and store until ready to eat.

PER SERVING Calories: 312 | Fat: 20 g | Protein: 23 g | Sodium: 665 mg | Fiber: 0 g | Carbohydrates: 7 g | Sugar: 4 g

Beef Ragu

This dish is divine on top of some cooked spaghetti squash. Add a pinch or two of freshly grated Parmesan cheese and you won't even miss the pasta. Keep this ragu in the refrigerator up to 1 week.

INGREDIENTS | SERVES 6

1 teaspoon olive oil

4 cloves garlic, minced

1½ pounds ground beef

1 teaspoon salt

1 teaspoon freshly ground pepper

1 teaspoon garlic powder

1 (14.5-ounce) can crushed tomatoes

¼ cup beef broth

2 teaspoons tomato paste

1 teaspoon dried thyme

2 bay leaves

1. Heat olive oil in a medium skillet over medium heat. Add garlic and cook until fragrant, about 2 minutes. Add ground beef, salt, pepper, and garlic powder and cook until beef is no longer pink, about 7 minutes.

2. Stir in remaining ingredients and bring to a simmer. Allow to simmer on the stove 20 minutes. Remove bay leaves.

3. Allow to cool and then divide into six equal portions. Store each portion in a separate airtight container in the refrigerator until ready to eat.

PER SERVING Calories: 222 | Fat: 12 g | Protein: 23 g | Sodium: 591 mg | Fiber: 2 g | Carbohydrates: 4 g | Sugar: 2 g

Taco Stuffed Zucchini Boats

The best way to reheat these zucchini boats is to bake them on 350°F for about 15 minutes and then turn your oven to broil for 2–3 minutes to crisp up the zucchini and the cheese a little bit. These boats will keep up to 1 week in your refrigerator.

INGREDIENTS | SERVES 6

3 large zucchini

1 tablespoon chili powder

1½ teaspoons cumin

½ teaspoon paprika

1 teaspoon salt

1 teaspoon freshly ground black pepper

¼ teaspoon dried oregano

¼ teaspoon crushed red pepper flakes

¼ teaspoon granulated garlic

¼ teaspoon granulated onion

1 tablespoon olive oil

½ cup diced red onion

1½ pounds ground beef

2 cups Enchilada Sauce (Chapter 9)

½ cup Mexican-blend shredded cheese

1. Preheat oven to 350°F. Cut each zucchini in half lengthwise and scoop out seeds to form wells. Set aside.

2. Combine spices in a small bowl and stir to mix well.

3. Heat olive oil in a medium skillet over medium heat and add onions. Cook until starting to soften, about 3 minutes. Add ground beef and spice mixture. Stir to combine and cook until beef is no longer pink, about 7 minutes.

4. Arrange zucchini cut side up in a single layer in a 9" × 13" baking dish. Scoop equal amounts of beef mixture into each zucchini well.

5. Pour enchilada sauce evenly over prepared zucchini and sprinkle cheese on top. Cover and bake 25 minutes. Uncover and bake 5 more minutes or until cheese starts to slightly brown.

6. Allow to cool and then transfer each zucchini boat to a separate airtight container. Store in the refrigerator until ready to eat.

PER SERVING   Calories: 258 | Fat: 14 g | Protein: 24 g | Sodium: 514 mg | Fiber: 3 g | Carbohydrates: 8 g | Sugar: 4 g

Mexican Stuffed Peppers

If you prefer to limit dairy, you can omit the cream cheese from this recipe. It lends a creamy texture to the beef, but you'll still end up with a flavor-packed stuffed pepper without it. You can keep these stuffed peppers in the refrigerator up to 1 week.

INGREDIENTS | SERVES 6

1 tablespoon chili powder

1½ teaspoons cumin

½ teaspoon paprika

1 teaspoon salt

1 teaspoon freshly ground black pepper

¼ teaspoon dried oregano

¼ teaspoon crushed red pepper flakes

¼ teaspoon granulated garlic

¼ teaspoon granulated onion

1 tablespoon olive oil

½ cup chopped yellow onion

1½ pounds ground beef

4 ounces cream cheese, cubed

½ cup shredded Cheddar cheese

½ cup shredded Monterey jack cheese

1 cup no-sugar-added salsa

6 medium green bell peppers, tops cut off and seeds removed

1. Preheat oven to 350°F.

2. Combine spices in a small bowl and stir to mix well.

3. Heat olive oil in a medium skillet over medium heat. Add onion and cook until starting to soften, about 3 minutes. Add beef and spice mixture and cook until beef is no longer pink, about 7 minutes.

4. Add cubed cream cheese to cooked beef and stir until cheese is melted and fully incorporated into beef. Stir in shredded cheeses and mix until melted.

5. Remove from heat and add salsa to beef and cheese. Mix well.

6. Scoop equal amounts of beef mixture into each pepper and place in a single layer in a 9" × 13" baking dish. Bake 30 minutes or until peppers have softened and mixture is hot and bubbly.

7. Allow to cool and then transfer to six separate airtight containers. Store in the refrigerator until you're ready to eat.

PER SERVING Calories: 407 | Fat: 27 g | Protein: 30 g | Sodium: 715 mg | Fiber: 3 g | Carbohydrates: 9 g | Sugar: 4 g

Different Color Peppers

All bell peppers come from the same species of plant (*Capsicum annuum*). The color of the pepper depends on when the pepper was harvested and how long it was allowed to ripen. Green bell peppers have been harvested before fully ripening. Yellow bell peppers are in the middle of ripening, and red bell peppers have been allowed to completely ripen. (That's why they're typically most expensive.) When it comes to nutrients, yellow and red peppers contain twice the vitamin C and almost nine times as much beta-carotene as their underripened counterpart.

Basil Meatballs

Freeze these meatballs for an hour (after cooking) in a single layer on a baking sheet, and then transfer them to an airtight container or a freezer bag. Freeze them in a single layer or they will mold together in a large clump, making them difficult to use later. The cooked meatballs will keep in the refrigerator up to 1 week.

INGREDIENTS | SERVES 6 (3 MEATBALLS PER SERVING)

1 cup fresh basil leaves

2 cloves garlic, minced

1 teaspoon lemon juice

1 teaspoon salt

¼ teaspoon freshly ground black pepper

¼ cup olive oil

3 tablespoons grated Parmesan cheese

1½ pounds ground beef

1 large egg

1. Preheat oven to 400°F and line a baking sheet with parchment paper.

2. Combine basil leaves, garlic, lemon juice, salt, and pepper in a food processor and process until broken up. With food processor running, slowly pour in olive oil and process until smooth. Add Parmesan cheese and pulse a few times to incorporate.

3. Transfer basil mixture to a medium bowl and add beef and egg. Mix with your hands until all ingredients are fully incorporated.

4. Form into eighteen meatballs and arrange in a single layer on prepared baking sheet. Bake 25 minutes or until cooked all the way through.

5. Allow meatballs to cool and then transfer three meatballs to each of six separate airtight containers. Store in the refrigerator until ready to eat.

PER SERVING Calories: 305 | Fat: 21 g | Protein: 24 g | Sodium: 530 mg | Fiber: 0 g | Carbohydrates: 1 g | Sugar: 0 g

Tamale Pie

Tamales are a traditional Mexican dish that incorporates meat wrapped in dough made of corn and then steamed in a corn husk. This low-carb take will give you all the traditional flavor without the high carbohydrate count. You can keep this dish in the refrigerator up to 1 week.

INGREDIENTS | SERVES 6

1 tablespoon olive oil

2 cloves garlic, minced

1 small yellow onion, peeled and diced

1½ pounds ground beef

1 teaspoon cumin

1 teaspoon chili powder

1 teaspoon salt

½ teaspoon freshly ground black pepper

1 large egg, whisked

½ cup Enchilada Sauce (Chapter 9)

½ cup shredded Monterey jack cheese

½ cup shredded Cheddar cheese

⅓ cup sour cream

1. Preheat oven to 350°F.

2. Heat olive oil in a medium skillet over medium heat and add garlic and onions; sauté until softened, about 4 minutes.

3. Add beef, cumin, chili powder, salt, and pepper and stir until meat is no longer pink, about 7 minutes. Remove from heat.

4. Transfer meat to a 9" × 13" baking pan. Add whisked egg and stir to thoroughly combine. Spread mixture evenly on the bottom of the pan.

5. Pour enchilada sauce on top of meat. Sprinkle cheeses over sauce. Use a spoon to dollop bits of sour cream all over the top.

6. Cover and bake 25 minutes. Uncover and bake another 5 minutes or until cheese is slightly browned.

7. Remove from oven and allow to cool. Divide into six equal portions and transfer each portion to a separate airtight container. Store in the refrigerator until ready to eat.

PER SERVING   Calories: 336 | Fat: 23 g | Protein: 28 g | Sodium: 622 mg | Fiber: 0.5 g | Carbohydrates: 2.5 g | Sugar: 1 g

Beef and Broccoli Alfredo

This recipe pairs really well with spaghetti squash. If you want to make a "pasta" meal out of it, put 1 cup cooked spaghetti squash in your container before putting prepared beef and broccoli into it. Mix it up thoroughly before eating. You can keep this dish in the refrigerator up to 1 week.

INGREDIENTS | SERVES 6

½ cup butter

8 ounces cream cheese

2 teaspoons garlic powder

2 cups full-fat coconut milk

1½ cups grated Parmesan cheese

¼ teaspoon freshly ground black pepper

1 tablespoon olive oil

1½ pounds ground beef

2 teaspoons granulated garlic

2 teaspoons granulated onion

1 teaspoon Italian seasoning

3 cups broccoli florets

Do You Have to Use Full-Fat Coconut Milk?

The full-fat coconut milk you get in a can is vastly different from the coconut milk beverages that are sold in a carton. In order to get the creamy texture of a traditional Alfredo sauce, you'll have to use the full-fat milk. The cans you're looking for are marked "original" instead of "lite" and can be found in the international aisle or the natural foods section of your grocery store.

1. Melt butter in a medium pan over medium heat. Add cream cheese and garlic powder and use a whisk to stir until cheese is melted and everything is smooth. Pour in coconut milk slowly, whisking the entire time. Stir in Parmesan cheese and mix until melted and smooth. Stir in pepper and remove from heat.

2. In a medium skillet, heat olive oil over medium heat, add ground beef, granulated garlic, granulated onion, and Italian seasoning and cook until beef is no longer pink, about 7 minutes.

3. Add broccoli to pan and cook 2 minutes to start softening. Turn heat to low, pour in prepared sauce, and cover. Allow to simmer until broccoli is soft but still a little crisp, about 5 minutes.

4. Remove from heat and allow to cool. Transfer six equal portions to separate airtight containers and store in the refrigerator until ready to eat.

PER SERVING Calories: 743 | Fat: 64 g | Protein: 34 g | Sodium: 674 mg | Fiber: 0.5 g | Carbohydrates: 9 g | Sugar: 1 g

Deconstructed Stuffed Mushrooms

If you want to add a little flavor and you're able to find nitrate-free, no-sugar-added bacon, add ¼ cup crumbled bacon to the skillet with the onions. You can keep this dish in the refrigerator for up to 1 week.

INGREDIENTS | SERVES 6

2 tablespoons olive oil

1 cup diced yellow onion

3 cups sliced white mushrooms

1½ pounds ground beef

2 tablespoons tomato paste

¼ cup beef broth

½ cup full-fat coconut milk

½ teaspoon arrowroot powder

1. Heat olive oil in a medium skillet over medium heat. Add onion and cook until softened, about 4 minutes. Add sliced mushrooms and cook 4 more minutes. Add beef and tomato paste and cook until beef is no longer pink, about 7 minutes.

2. Add beef broth and stir. Turn heat to high and bring to a boil. Reduce heat to medium and allow to simmer 5 minutes. Reduce heat to low and stir in coconut milk and arrowroot powder. Stir constantly until mixture thickens, about 2 minutes.

3. Remove from heat and allow to cool. Divide into six equal portions and transfer each portion to a separate airtight container. Store in the refrigerator until ready to eat.

PER SERVING Calories: 311 | Fat: 20 g | Protein: 25 g | Sodium: 159 mg | Fiber: 2.5 g | Carbohydrates: 8 g | Sugar: 4 g

Spicy Beef and Peppers

This recipe comes together in minutes, and once it's done cooking in the slow cooker, you have a hearty protein source for six of your meals. You can keep this in the refrigerator up to 1 week.

INGREDIENTS | SERVES 6

½ teaspoon paprika

½ teaspoon granulated garlic

½ teaspoon salt

½ teaspoon freshly ground black pepper

1 (2-pound) chuck roast

5 cloves garlic, roughly chopped

1 small white onion, peeled and sliced

1 cup beef broth

1 (12-ounce) jar sliced pepperoncini peppers

1. Combine spices in a small bowl and stir to mix well. Coat chuck roast in spices, covering as much as you can.

2. Put garlic and onions in the bottom of slow cooker, add roast on top, and pour in beef broth and contents of pepperoncini jar (peppers and liquid).

3. Cook on low 6 hours or until beef is tender. Shred beef with two forks.

4. Divide beef and peppers evenly among six airtight containers. Store in the refrigerator until ready to eat.

PER SERVING Calories: 264 | Fat: 10 g | Protein: 33 g | Sodium: 428 mg | Fiber: 1 g | Carbohydrates: 7 g | Sugar: 3 g

Pepperoncini versus Banana Peppers

Pepperoncini and banana peppers are two of the mildest peppers you can get. They're extremely similar in both taste and look; the only major difference is their heat factor. Pepperoncini range from 100 to 500 SHU (the unit of measure for pepper heat), while banana peppers range from 0 to 500. For comparison, jalapeño peppers range from 2,500 to 5,000 SHU. Because pepperoncini and banana peppers are so similar, you can use them interchangeably in most recipes.

Italian Meatball Bake

This is another recipe that goes exceptionally well with cooked spaghetti squash. You can also pair it with basic Cauliflower "Rice" (Chapter 13). You can keep these meatballs in the refrigerator up to 1 week.

INGREDIENTS | SERVES 6

1½ pounds ground beef
¼ cup unblanched almond flour
½ cup shredded zucchini, strained
3 large eggs, divided
1 tablespoon dried parsley
1 teaspoon salt
¼ teaspoon granulated garlic
¼ teaspoon granulated onion
¼ teaspoon dried oregano
¼ cup grated Parmesan cheese
2 cups no-sugar-added marinara sauce
2 cups mozzarella cheese

1. Preheat oven to 375°F.

2. Combine beef, almond flour, zucchini, 2 eggs, parsley, salt, garlic, onion, oregano, and Parmesan cheese in a medium bowl. Mix with your hands until thoroughly combined. Form into eighteen meatballs and arrange in a single layer on a baking sheet lined with parchment paper.

3. Bake 20 minutes, flipping meatballs once during cooking.

4. After meatballs are cooked, transfer them to a 9" × 13" baking dish and pour marinara sauce on top. Whisk remaining egg and pour on top of meatballs and sauce. Stir to incorporate and spread meatballs out evenly. Sprinkle with mozzarella cheese.

5. Bake 30 minutes or until cheese is bubbly and starts to brown. Remove from oven and allow to cool.

6. Divide into six equal portions and store each portion in an airtight container in the refrigerator until ready to eat.

PER SERVING   Calories: 403 | Fat: 25 g | Protein: 36 g | Sodium: 811 mg | Fiber: 25 g | Carbohydrates: 6 g | Sugar: 2 g

Ground Beef Hash

This recipe is great at any time of the day. If you have a little extra time for some additional prep, poach an egg or two right before eating and put them on top. You can keep this hash in the refrigerator up to 1 week.

INGREDIENTS | SERVES 6

4 tablespoons avocado oil
2 cups roughly chopped cauliflower
¼ cup chopped yellow onion
1 tablespoon minced jalapeño
1½ pounds ground beef
1 teaspoon granulated garlic
1 teaspoon granulated onion
1 teaspoon salt
1 teaspoon freshly ground black pepper
½ teaspoon dried parsley
1½ cups pepper jack cheese

Be Aware of Smoke Points

This recipe calls for avocado oil because it's more stable at higher temperatures than olive oil. If you don't have avocado oil, it's best to swap it out with ghee or butter instead. Cooking olive oil at too high a temperature can cause the oil to burn, creating by-products that aren't good for you. The point at which an oil or fat starts to burn is called its smoke point.

1. Heat avocado oil in a medium skillet over high heat. Allow oil to get really hot, then add cauliflower. Stir once to coat, then let cauliflower sit undisturbed 2 minutes, watching closely to make sure it doesn't burn. Stir again and then let cauliflower sit 2 more minutes.

2. Turn heat down to medium and add onions and jalapeños. Cook until softened, about 4 minutes. Add beef, spices, and herbs and cook until meat is no longer pink, about 7 minutes.

3. Remove from heat and stir in cheese until melted.

4. Allow to cool and then divide into six equal portions. Transfer each portion to a separate airtight container and store in the refrigerator until ready to eat.

PER SERVING Calories: 427 | Fat: 31 g | Protein: 31 g | Sodium: 685 mg | Fiber: 1 g | Carbohydrates: 4 g | Sugar: 1 g

Carne Asada

It takes less than 20 minutes to prepare this dish, but the recipe requires you to marinate the steak at least 2 hours. Keep that in mind when designing your meal plan and plan your prep days accordingly. You can keep this meat in the refrigerator up to 1 week.

INGREDIENTS | SERVES 6

3 cloves garlic, minced

½ cup coconut aminos

1 cup chopped fresh cilantro

½ teaspoon salt

¼ teaspoon freshly ground black pepper

¼ cup olive oil

2 tablespoons apple cider vinegar

Juice of 2 medium limes, about 4 tablespoons

1 fresh medium jalapeño, seeded and minced

1½ pounds flank steak

1. Combine all ingredients except steak in a gallon-sized zip-top bag. Seal tightly and shake or massage bag to mix well.

2. Add steak to bag and massage again to make sure all meat is covered in marinade. Allow to sit in the refrigerator 2 hours or overnight.

3. Heat grill to high heat and cook steak 8 minutes. Flip steak over and cook another 8 minutes or until steak reaches desired level of doneness.

4. Remove from grill and allow meat to rest 10 minutes. Cut into strips and divide into six equal portions. Transfer each portion to a separate airtight container and store in the refrigerator until ready to eat.

PER SERVING Calories: 277 | Fat: 17 g | Protein: 25 g | Sodium: 615 mg | Fiber: 0 g | Carbohydrates: 4 g | Sugar: 1 g

Pizza Meatballs

When that pizza craving strikes, reach for these meatballs instead. They provide all the same flavor and cheesy goodness with significantly fewer carbs. These meatballs will keep in the refrigerator up to 1 week.

INGREDIENTS | SERVES 6 (3 MEATBALLS PER SERVING)

1½ pounds ground beef

1 cup unblanched almond flour

1 large egg

1 teaspoon garlic salt

2 teaspoons minced dried onion

1 teaspoon Italian seasoning

1 (6-ounce) block mozzarella cheese, cut into 18 cubes

3 (14-ounce) jars no-sugar-added pizza sauce

1 teaspoon dried basil

½ teaspoon dried oregano

Basic Pizza Sauce

If you can't find a jarred or canned pizza sauce with ingredients that you like, you can easily make your own. Combine 2 (15-ounce) cans of no-sugar-added tomato sauce, 1 (8-ounce) can of tomato paste, 1 tablespoon dried oregano, 1½ tablespoons dried minced garlic, 1 teaspoon paprika, ½ teaspoon onion powder, and 1½ teaspoons dried basil in a blender or food processor and process until smooth.

1. Preheat oven to 400°F.

2. Combine ground beef, almond flour, egg, garlic salt, onion, and Italian seasoning in a large bowl and mix until thoroughly combined. Shape into 18 meatballs and set on a baking sheet lined with parchment paper.

3. Push a cube of mozzarella cheese into the center of each meatball and reshape to make sure cheese is completely covered.

4. Bake 20 minutes and remove from oven. (Meatballs don't have to be fully cooked.)

5. Combine pizza sauce, basil, and oregano in a large saucepan. Add meatballs and stir. Bring to a simmer over low heat.

6. Allow to simmer 20–25 minutes or until meatballs are fully cooked and flavors are developed.

7. Divide into six equal portions and put each portion in a separate airtight container. Store in the refrigerator until ready to eat.

PER SERVING   Calories: 400 | Fat: 27 g | Protein: 33 g | Sodium: 649 mg | Fiber: 2 g | Carbohydrates: 5 g | Sugar: 1 g

Taco Salad

Storing the lettuce in its own bag helps keep it crisp until you're ready to eat your taco salad. If you prefer a wilted lettuce, skip this step and add the lettuce directly to the beef mixture when tossing to combine. You can keep this in the refrigerator up to 1 week.

INGREDIENTS | SERVES 6

1 tablespoon chili powder

1½ teaspoons cumin

½ teaspoon paprika

1 teaspoon salt

1 teaspoon freshly ground black pepper

¼ teaspoon dried oregano

¼ teaspoon crushed red pepper flakes

¼ teaspoon granulated garlic

¼ teaspoon granulated onion

1 tablespoon olive oil

1½ pounds ground beef

1½ cups chopped cherry tomatoes

½ cup shredded Cheddar cheese

1½ cups no-sugar-added salsa

1½ cups sour cream

6 tablespoons chopped scallions

6 cups chopped romaine lettuce

1. Combine spices in a small bowl and stir to mix well. Heat olive oil in a medium skillet over medium heat and add ground beef and spice mixture. Cook until beef is no longer pink, about 7 minutes.

2. Remove from heat and allow to cool completely.

3. In a separate medium bowl, combine all remaining ingredients except lettuce. Toss to combine. When beef has cooled, add to bowl and toss to incorporate.

4. Divide beef mixture into six equal portions and place each portion in an airtight container. Put 1 cup shredded lettuce into each of six sandwich bags and seal tightly. Place one lettuce-filled bag in each container and secure lid in place. Store in the refrigerator.

5. When ready to eat, add lettuce to beef mixture and toss to combine.

PER SERVING   Calories: 390 | Fat: 27 g | Protein: 27 g | Sodium: 984 mg | Fiber: 2.5 g | Carbohydrates: 9 g | Sugar: 5 g

Meatball Zoodle Soup

Instead of using your slow cooker, add all ingredients except zucchini and cooked meatballs to your pressure cooker. Turn on the Soup setting and cook on high for 10 minutes. Stir in zucchini noodles while soup is still hot. You can keep the completed soup in the refrigerator up to 1 week.

INGREDIENTS | SERVES 6

1½ pounds ground beef
¼ cup unblanched almond flour
4 cloves garlic, minced
1 large egg
2 teaspoons salt, divided
½ teaspoon freshly ground black pepper
1 teaspoon minced dried onion
2 teaspoons dried parsley
6 cups beef broth
1 tablespoon coconut aminos
3 stalks celery, diced
1 small yellow onion, peeled and diced
1 large tomato, seeded and diced
1 teaspoon granulated garlic
2 large zucchini, spiralized

Spiralizing Your Vegetables

In order to effectively spiralize your zucchini, you'll need a special cutting tool called a spiralizer. If you don't have one or prefer not to get one, you can julienne the zucchini instead. You will lose the noodle effect, but you won't sacrifice any flavor.

1. Preheat oven to 400°F.

2. Combine beef, almond flour, garlic, egg, 1 teaspoon salt, pepper, onion, and parsley in a medium bowl. Mix with your hands until fully incorporated. Form into twenty-four meatballs.

3. Arrange meatballs on a baking sheet lined with parchment paper. Bake 12 minutes, rotating meatballs once during cooking. It's okay if meatballs are not cooked through.

4. Combine remaining ingredients except zucchini in slow cooker and add meatballs. Cook on low 6 hours. After 6 hours, turn slow cooker off and stir in spiralized zucchini. It will soften from the heat of the soup.

5. Allow to cool and then divide into six equal portions, transferring each portion to an airtight container. Store in the refrigerator until ready to eat.

PER SERVING Calories: 294 | Fat: 15 g | Protein: 29 g | Sodium: 1,563 mg | Fiber: 3 g | Carbohydrates: 9 g | Sugar: 5 g

Greek Meatball Salad

Instead of making this a salad, you can use large iceberg lettuce leaves to wrap up meatballs with chopped tomatoes, chopped cucumbers, and Tzatziki Sauce (Chapter 9) and make lettuce wraps. You can store this in the refrigerator up to 1 week.

INGREDIENTS | SERVES 6

½ cup finely chopped white onion
1 tablespoon Greek seasoning
½ teaspoon garlic powder
¼ teaspoon ground cumin
1½ pounds ground beef
1½ cups chopped cherry tomatoes
1½ cups chopped cucumber
1½ cups Tzatziki Sauce (Chapter 9)
6 cups chopped iceberg lettuce

Homemade Greek Seasoning

If you don't have ready-made Greek seasoning, you can make your own by combining 2 teaspoons salt, 1 teaspoon freshly ground black pepper, 2 teaspoons granulated garlic, 2 teaspoons dried basil, 2 teaspoons dried oregano, 1 teaspoon dried parsley, 1 teaspoon dried rosemary, 1 teaspoon dried dill, 1 teaspoon dried marjoram, ½ teaspoon dried thyme, 1 teaspoon ground cinnamon, and ½ teaspoon ground nutmeg in an airtight container and mixing well. Use what you need and then store the rest in a cool, dry place for later.

1. Preheat oven to 400°F.

2. Combine onions, Greek seasoning, garlic powder, cumin, and beef in a large bowl. Mix with your hands until everything is fully incorporated. Form into twenty-four meatballs.

3. Arrange meatballs on a baking sheet lined with parchment paper and bake 20 minutes, turning meatballs once during cooking.

4. Put four meatballs in each of six airtight containers. Add ¼ cup tomatoes, ¼ cup cucumbers, and ¼ cup Tzatziki Sauce to each container.

5. Put 1 cup chopped lettuce into each of six sandwich bags and seal tightly. Place one lettuce-filled bag in each container and secure lid in place. Store in the refrigerator.

6. When ready to eat, add lettuce to meatballs and toss to combine.

PER SERVING Calories: 261 | Fat: 13 g | Protein: 25 g | Sodium: 112 mg | Fiber: 2 g | Carbohydrates: 9 g | Sugar: 6 g

Philly Cheese Steak Zucchini Boats

If you like your zucchini crunchy and want to save some time, you can forgo the baking and eat these boats right after you fill them with the cooked Philly cheese steak mixture. These boats will store in the refrigerator up to 1 week.

INGREDIENTS | SERVES 6

6 large zucchini
2 tablespoons ghee
1 small yellow onion, peeled and diced
8 ounces white mushrooms, diced
1½ pounds ground beef
1 teaspoon salt
1 teaspoon freshly ground black pepper
1 teaspoon granulated garlic
1 tablespoon coconut aminos
2 tablespoons tomato paste
8 ounces provolone cheese, sliced

1. Preheat oven to 350°F. Cut each zucchini in half lengthwise and scoop out seeds to form wells. Arrange zucchini cut side up in a 9" × 13" baking dish.

2. Heat ghee over medium-high heat in a medium skillet. Add onion and cook until softened, about 4 minutes. Add mushrooms and cook another 3 minutes. Add beef, salt, pepper, and granulated garlic and cook until beef is no longer pink, about 7 minutes.

3. Stir in coconut aminos and tomato paste and allow to simmer 1 minute. Place cheese slices on top and cover, allowing steam to melt cheese, about 3 minutes. Stir to incorporate cheese into beef.

4. Remove from heat and divide into six equal portions. Scoop each portion into the well of a prepared zucchini.

5. Bake 20 minutes or until zucchini is softened but still slightly crisp. Allow to cool and then transfer each zucchini boat to a separate airtight container. Store in the refrigerator until ready to eat.

PER SERVING   Calories: 444 | Fat: 26 g | Protein: 37 g | Sodium: 931 mg | Fiber: 5 g | Carbohydrates: 15 g | Sugar: 10 g

Beef and Cabbage Casserole

This recipe requires only one pot, which makes both cooking and cleanup a breeze. You can keep this casserole in the refrigerator up to 1 week.

INGREDIENTS | SERVES 6

1 tablespoon olive oil

1 medium yellow onion, peeled and chopped

1½ pounds ground beef

1 teaspoon salt

1 teaspoon freshly ground black pepper

½ teaspoon paprika

3 cups roughly chopped cabbage

1½ cups riced cauliflower

1 (8-ounce) can no-sugar-added tomato sauce

1 (14-ounce) can petite diced tomatoes

2 cups beef broth

1 cup shredded Cheddar cheese

1. Heat olive oil in a medium skillet over medium heat and add onions. Cook until softened, about 3 minutes. Add beef, salt, pepper, and paprika and cook until no longer pink, about 7 minutes.

2. Add remaining ingredients except cheese and stir to combine. Cover and allow to simmer 20 minutes or until cabbage and cauliflower are soft.

3. Sprinkle cheese on top and continue cooking covered, about 4 minutes or until cheese is fully melted.

4. Allow to cool and then divide into six equal portions. Transfer each portion to a separate airtight container and store in the refrigerator until ready to eat.

PER SERVING Calories: 536 | Fat: 30 g | Protein: 53 g | Sodium: 997 mg | Fiber: 4 g | Carbohydrates: 10 g | Sugar: 6 g

Stock Up on Cauliflower Rice

You used to have no other option but to rice your own cauliflower, but with the increasing popularity of low-carb and Paleo diets came an increased availability of store-bought riced cauliflower. If you want to save yourself some time, check your grocery store's frozen or refrigerated food section to see if it has riced cauliflower available. If it does, you can stock up when there's a sale and keep it in your freezer to use quickly in recipes like this whenever you need it.

Cheeseburger Meatloaf

Cooking the garlic and onions before adding them to the meatloaf helps develop the flavors a bit, but if you want to save some time during your meal prep, you can add them to the beef mixture without that extra step. You can keep the cooked meatloaf in the refrigerator up to 1 week.

INGREDIENTS | SERVES 6

1 tablespoon olive oil

3 cloves garlic, minced

¼ cup minced yellow onion

1½ pounds ground beef

¾ cup almond meal

2 large eggs, beaten

1 teaspoon salt

1 teaspoon freshly ground black pepper

2 teaspoons coconut aminos

2 cups shredded Cheddar cheese

⅓ cup Ketchup (Chapter 9)

¼ cup mustard

1. Heat avocado oil in a medium skillet over medium heat. Add garlic and onion and cook until softened, about 3 minutes. Transfer to a large bowl.

2. Add ground beef, almond meal, eggs, salt, pepper, and coconut aminos to the onion mixture and mix thoroughly to combine. Spread beef out in a flat rectangle and sprinkle cheese on top.

3. Shape into a meatloaf by lifting sides to fully cover cheese and then pressing beef together.

4. Transfer to a 9" × 5" loaf pan and spread ketchup and mustard on top.

5. Bake 1 hour or until beef is fully cooked through. Allow to cool and then divide into six equal portions. Transfer each portion to a separate airtight container and store in the refrigerator until ready to eat.

PER SERVING   Calories: 528 | Fat: 37 g | Protein: 38 g | Sodium: 967 mg | Fiber: 2 g | Carbohydrates: 10 g | Sugar: 4 g

Beef Stir-Fry

This dish goes very well with cauliflower rice or zucchini noodles. If you want to pair it with spiralized zucchini, cooking the zucchini is not necessary. Just scoop hot beef and sauce over the raw noodles, and they will soften a bit. This stir-fry will keep in the refrigerator up to 1 week.

INGREDIENTS | SERVES 6

2 tablespoons avocado oil

5 cloves garlic, chopped

1½ pounds ground beef

1 teaspoon salt

1 teaspoon freshly ground black pepper

½ teaspoon Chinese five spice

1 cup shredded green cabbage

1 large red bell pepper, seeded and sliced

1 large orange bell pepper, seeded and sliced

2 tablespoons coconut aminos

1 teaspoon arrowroot powder

¼ cup beef broth

What Is Chinese Five Spice?

Chinese five spice is a combination of at least five spices that are meant to satisfy all five of your taste senses—bitter, sweet, sour, salty, and umami (also described as pungent or savory). It typically contains star anise, cloves, cinnamon, fennel, and Szechuan pepper. You can purchase Chinese five spice in the spice section at most supermarkets.

1. Heat avocado oil in a wok or medium skillet over medium-high heat. Add garlic and cook until fragrant, about 2 minutes. Add ground beef, salt, pepper, and Chinese five spice and cook until beef is no longer pink, about 7 minutes.

2. Add cabbage and bell peppers and cook until vegetables are tender, about 5 minutes.

3. Add coconut aminos and stir. Stir arrowroot powder into beef broth and stir into beef mixture.

4. Continue to cook, stirring frequently, until sauce has thickened, about 4 minutes.

5. Remove from heat and allow to cool. Divide into six equal portions and transfer each portion to a separate airtight container. Store in the refrigerator until ready to eat.

PER SERVING Calories: 266 | Fat: 15 g | Protein: 23 g | Sodium: 648 mg | Fiber: 2 g | Carbohydrates: 6 g | Sugar: 3 g

CHAPTER 6

Pork

BBQ Shredded Pork

If you want to save some time, you can skip the second step and add peppered pork directly to the slow cooker without browning. The browning process increases depth of flavor, but the end result is still delicious without it. This pork can last in the refrigerator up to 1 week.

INGREDIENTS | SERVES 6

1½ teaspoons freshly ground black pepper

1½ pounds pork butt

2 tablespoons olive oil

1 (14-ounce) can beef broth

2 cups Basic Barbecue Sauce (Chapter 9)

Choosing Pork Wisely

Pork butt is a less expensive cut of meat, but it does have a higher fat content than more expensive cuts like pork tenderloin. More than 90 percent of the pesticides Americans consume are found in the fat and tissue of meat and dairy products, since toxins are stored in fat. It's especially important to choose organic or responsibly raised meats when using fattier cuts.

1. Rub pork with black pepper, covering as much as possible.

2. Heat olive oil in a large skillet over medium heat. Add pork butt and cook 1–2 minutes on each side. You don't have to cook pork; just brown it.

3. Transfer browned pork to a slow cooker and pour in beef broth. Cook on low 8 hours or until pork pulls apart easily with a fork.

4. Remove pork, shred with two forks, and drain excess liquid. Transfer shredded pork back to slow cooker and stir in barbecue sauce. Cook on high 1 hour.

5. Divide pork into six equal portions and store each portion in an airtight container until ready to eat.

PER SERVING Calories: 343 | Fat: 15 g | Protein: 26 g | Sodium: 948 mg | Fiber: 1 g | Carbohydrates: 15 g | Sugar: 3 g

Italian Sausage and Roasted Veggies

This recipe is extremely easy to make, and it's a complete meal all by itself. You can prepare it as written or use your favorite low-carb vegetable combo. This dish will last up to 1 week in the refrigerator.

INGREDIENTS | SERVES 6

2 tablespoons Italian seasoning

½ teaspoon granulated garlic

½ teaspoon granulated onion

¼ teaspoon crushed red pepper flakes

2 cups peeled and cubed turnips

2 medium zucchini, cut into medallions

2 cups broccoli florets, cut into bite-sized pieces

1 cup cauliflower florets, cut into bite-sized pieces

1 large red bell pepper, seeded and sliced into thin strips

1 large orange bell pepper, seeded and sliced into thin strips

1½ pounds no-sugar-added Italian sausage, cut into medallions

3 tablespoons olive oil

1. Preheat oven to 400°F.

2. Combine Italian seasoning, granulated garlic, granulated onion, and red pepper flakes in a small bowl.

3. Place vegetables and Italian sausage in a large bowl and toss to combine.

4. Spread vegetables and sausage out in a single layer on a baking sheet lined with parchment paper. Pour oil on top and toss to coat, then spread out again.

5. Sprinkle seasoning mixture over vegetables and sausage.

6. Roast 15 minutes, flip vegetables and sausage over, and roast another 15 minutes or until vegetables are tender but still crisp and sausage is cooked.

7. Divide into six equal portions, place each portion in an airtight container, and store in the refrigerator until ready to eat.

PER SERVING   Calories: 434 | Fat: 35 g | Protein: 20 g | Sodium: 820 mg | Fiber: 4 g | Carbohydrates: 12 g | Sugar: 7 g

Breakfast Sausage

If you want to freeze this breakfast sausage and cook it as you go, shape it into patties, freeze in a single layer on a baking sheet 1 hour, and then transfer to an airtight container or freezer bag. You can keep them frozen up to 6 months. The cooked patties will keep 1 week in the refrigerator.

INGREDIENTS | SERVES 6 (2 PATTIES PER SERVING)

1 teaspoon dried sage

1½ teaspoons fennel seeds

1½ teaspoons salt

¼ teaspoon dried marjoram

¼ teaspoon crushed red pepper flakes

1½ pounds ground pork

1 tablespoon olive oil

1. Combine spices and herbs in a medium bowl and stir to mix well. Add pork and use your hands to incorporate spices into pork mixture. Shape into twelve patties.

2. Heat olive oil in a medium pan over medium heat. Add patties in a single layer and cook 5 minutes on each side or until pork is cooked through and outside is browned.

3. Transfer two patties to each of six airtight containers and store in the refrigerator until ready to eat.

PER SERVING Calories: 314 | Fat: 25 g | Protein: 19 g | Sodium: 644 mg | Fiber: 0 g | Carbohydrates: 0 g | Sugar: 0 g

Pulled Pork Chili

This recipe is so simple, you can have it ready to go in under 10 minutes. All you have to do is combine everything in a slow cooker and then come back to it when it's done cooking and enjoy. This chili will keep 1 week in the refrigerator.

INGREDIENTS | SERVES 6

1½ pounds pork shoulder

1 small yellow onion, peeled and diced

1 medium jalapeño, seeded and diced

1 (15-ounce) can petite diced tomatoes

1 (15-ounce) can fire-roasted tomatoes

1 (4.5-ounce) can green chilies

1 (8-ounce) can no-sugar-added tomato sauce

2 teaspoons chili powder

1 teaspoon cumin

½ teaspoon paprika

1 teaspoon granulated garlic

½ teaspoon dried cilantro

1 cup no-sugar-added chicken broth

1. Combine all ingredients in a slow cooker. Stir to mix well.

2. Cook on low 7 hours or until pork shreds easily with a fork. Remove pork from chili and shred with two forks. Return pork to slow cooker and stir to combine.

3. Divide into six equal portions and store each portion in an airtight container until ready to eat.

PER SERVING Calories: 221 | Fat: 9 g | Protein: 25 g | Sodium: 463 mg | Fiber: 4 g | Carbohydrates: 11 g | Sugar: 6 g

Pork Stir-Fry

This dish is a complete meal as is, but if you want to add a different texture, you can combine it with ½ cup cauliflower rice. This stir-fry should keep in the refrigerator up to 1 week.

INGREDIENTS | SERVES 6

1½ pounds ground pork

1 teaspoon salt

½ teaspoon freshly ground black pepper

½ cup apple cider vinegar

⅓ cup Ketchup (Chapter 9)

1 tablespoon coconut aminos

1 large yellow onion, peeled and sliced

1 medium yellow bell pepper, seeded and sliced

2 cups broccoli florets, cut into bite-sized pieces

With the Mother

When choosing an apple cider vinegar, opt for one that contains "the mother." The mother is a combination of acids and bacteria that are responsible for most of the vinegar's health benefits. Vinegars without the mother have been refined and processed and stripped of important nutrients. You'll be able to identify apple cider vinegar with the mother because it looks cloudy and murky with sediment floating around rather than clear.

1. Heat pork in a medium skillet over medium heat. Add salt and pepper and cook until pork is no longer pink, about 7 minutes. Drain excess grease.

2. While pork is cooking, combine vinegar, ketchup, and coconut aminos in a small bowl and stir to mix well.

3. Add vegetables to skillet and stir until starting to soften but still crisp, about 3 minutes.

4. Pour vinegar mixture over pork and vegetables and cover. Reduce heat to medium-low and allow to cook until vegetables are tender, about 5 minutes.

5. Divide into six equal portions and put each portion in an airtight container. Store in the refrigerator until ready to eat.

PER SERVING Calories: 341 | Fat: 23 g | Protein: 20 g | Sodium: 672 mg | Fiber: 2 g | Carbohydrates: 10 g | Sugar: 5 g

Sausage Muffins

Don't let the name of this recipe fool you; these "muffins" are made from coconut flour and eggs, so they're low-carb and gluten-free. They're also extremely portable, making them an ideal choice for meal prep. They'll last up to 1 week in the refrigerator.

INGREDIENTS | SERVES 6 (2 MUFFINS PER SERVING)

1 tablespoon olive oil

1½ pounds ground no-sugar-added sausage

½ cup chopped spinach

½ teaspoon baking powder

1 teaspoon garlic powder

½ cup coconut flour

½ teaspoon salt

6 large eggs, beaten

6 tablespoons butter, melted

1. Preheat oven to 400°F and line a 12-cup muffin tin with cupcake liners (or grease the pan).

2. Heat olive oil in a medium skillet over medium heat. Add sausage and cook until no longer pink, about 7 minutes. Add spinach and cook until wilted, about 2 more minutes. Remove from heat.

3. In a medium bowl, combine baking powder, garlic powder, coconut flour, and salt. Stir to mix well. Stir in eggs and butter. Fold in sausage and stir to combine.

4. Pour equal amounts of mixture into each muffin well. Bake 20 minutes or until biscuits have set.

5. Remove from oven and allow to cool. Place two muffins in each of six airtight containers and store in the refrigerator until ready to eat.

PER SERVING   Calories: 534 | Fat: 47 g | Protein: 25 g | Sodium: 932 mg | Fiber: 6 g | Carbohydrates: 8.5 g | Sugar: 1 g

Pork Roast and Sauerkraut

If you want to kick this roast up a notch, you can add some sliced Italian sausage to the sauerkraut before cooking. Be sure to choose a sausage without any artificial ingredients or sugar, or better yet, make your own! You can keep this dish in the refrigerator up to 1 week.

INGREDIENTS | SERVES 6

2 tablespoons olive oil

1½ pounds pork tenderloin

1 teaspoon dried thyme

1 teaspoon salt

¼ teaspoon freshly ground black pepper

3 (14.5-ounce) cans sauerkraut

1 tablespoon caraway seeds

What Is Sauerkraut?

Sauerkraut is finely sliced cabbage that has been fermented for a period of 4–6 weeks. The fermentation process makes sauerkraut one of the best probiotic-rich foods you can eat. The consumption of probiotic-rich foods has been shown to contribute to digestive health, help with weight loss, balance mood, and improve immune system function.

1. Preheat oven broiler.

2. Brush olive oil all over pork tenderloin and sprinkle with thyme, salt, and pepper. Transfer pork loin to a baking sheet and cook under broiler 10 minutes, turning once while cooking.

3. Add sauerkraut to a slow cooker and sprinkle with caraway seeds. Stir to combine. Place browned pork loin on top of sauerkraut.

4. Cook on low 6 hours or until pork comes apart easily with a fork. Remove pork from slow cooker and shred with two forks. Return pork to slow cooker and stir to combine.

5. Divide into six equal portions and transfer each portion to a separate airtight container. Store in the refrigerator until ready to eat.

PER SERVING Calories: 201 | Fat: 7 g | Protein: 25 g | Sodium: 1,233 mg | Fiber: 6 g | Carbohydrates: 9 g | Sugar: 3 g

Italian Meatballs

Combine these meatballs with cooked spaghetti squash or zucchini noodles and a little bit of marinara sauce, and you have a fully balanced low-carb meal. These Italian meatballs will keep in the refrigerator up to 6 days.

INGREDIENTS | SERVES 6

1½ pounds ground pork

⅓ cup almond meal

2 large eggs, beaten

2 cloves garlic, minced

1 tablespoon minced dried onion

¼ cup chopped fresh parsley

1 teaspoon salt

½ teaspoon freshly ground black pepper

1 teaspoon Italian seasoning

2 tablespoons grated Parmesan cheese

1. Preheat oven to 425°F.

2. Combine all ingredients in a large bowl and mix well. Shape mixture into eighteen equal-sized meatballs and arrange meatballs in a single layer on a baking sheet.

3. Bake 20 minutes or until meatballs are browned and fully cooked through, turning meatballs once during cooking.

4. Transfer three meatballs to each of six airtight containers and store in the refrigerator until ready to eat.

PER SERVING Calories: 366 | Fat: 29 g | Protein: 23 g | Sodium: 513 mg | Fiber: 1 g | Carbohydrates: 2.5 g | Sugar: 0 g

Balsamic Pork Tenderloin

Cauliflower Mash (Chapter 10) and Mozzarella and Basil Tomatoes (Chapter 10) make great side dishes for this pork. Consider planning your meals for the week to include all three so you can enjoy them together. This pork will last up to 1 week in the refrigerator.

INGREDIENTS | SERVES 6

2 cloves garlic, minced

2 tablespoons steak seasoning

½ cup olive oil

⅓ cup balsamic vinegar

1½ pounds pork tenderloin

1. Combine garlic, steak seasoning, olive oil, and balsamic vinegar in a gallon-sized bag and massage to mix well. Add pork tenderloin and massage to cover pork. Seal and allow pork to marinate 2 hours or overnight.

2. Preheat oven to 350°F.

3. Transfer pork and marinade to a 9" × 13" baking dish and bake 1 hour, basting pork every 15 minutes. Remove from oven and allow to rest 10 minutes.

4. Slice pork and transfer equal portions to each of six airtight containers. Store in the refrigerator until ready to eat.

PER SERVING Calories: 295 | Fat: 20 g | Protein: 23 g | Sodium: 63 mg | Fiber: 0 g | Carbohydrates: 3 g | Sugar: 2 g

Roasted Pork Loin

You can also cook this in your slow cooker by adding ¼ cup chicken broth to a slow cooker, along with the seasoned pork, and cooking 6 hours on low. This will keep up to 1 week in the refrigerator.

INGREDIENTS | SERVES 6

1 teaspoon granulated garlic

2 teaspoons dried rosemary

½ teaspoon dried sage

1 teaspoon salt

½ teaspoon freshly ground black pepper

1½ pounds pork tenderloin

¼ cup olive oil

1. Preheat oven to 350°F.

2. Combine spices in a small bowl and stir to mix well. Rub spices all over meat, covering as much as possible.

3. Transfer pork to a large roasting pan and lightly brush olive oil on top, using care not to brush off spices.

4. Roast 45 minutes or until pork is cooked through, basting roast with pan juices every 15 minutes.

5. Remove from oven and allow to cool. Cut into twelve slices and transfer two slices to each of six separate airtight containers. Store in the refrigerator until ready to eat.

PER SERVING   Calories: 205 | Fat: 11 g | Protein: 23 g | Sodium: 447 mg | Fiber: 0 g | Carbohydrates: 1 g | Sugar: 0 g

Spicy Pork Tenderloin

If you prefer to make this pork tenderloin indoors, you can bake in a 325°F oven 40–45 minutes, turning over halfway, until pork is cooked through and tender. This cooked tenderloin will keep in the refrigerator up to 1 week.

INGREDIENTS | SERVES 6

2 tablespoons chili powder

1 teaspoon paprika

1 teaspoon salt

¼ teaspoon dried thyme

¼ teaspoon ground ginger

½ teaspoon garlic powder

¼ teaspoon freshly ground black pepper

1½ pounds pork tenderloin

2 tablespoons olive oil

1. Combine spices in a small bowl and stir to mix well.

2. Rub dry spice mixture all over tenderloin, covering as much of the surface as you can. Wrap tenderloin tightly in plastic wrap and refrigerate 3 hours to let flavors develop.

3. Preheat grill to medium heat. Brush olive oil on grill grate and grill tenderloin 40 minutes, turning during cooking process to cook evenly.

4. Cut tenderloin into twelve slices and put two slices into each of six airtight containers. Store in the refrigerator until ready to eat.

PER SERVING   Calories: 172 | Fat: 8 g | Protein: 23 g | Sodium: 524 mg | Fiber: 1 g | Carbohydrates: 2 g | Sugar: 0 g

Pork and Cauliflower Rice Skillet Meal

The best way to reheat this skillet meal is by adding a little olive oil to a medium pan and cooking over low heat until everything is heated through. This meal will keep up to 1 week in the refrigerator.

INGREDIENTS | SERVES 6

3 tablespoons olive oil

2 cloves garlic, minced

1 large yellow onion, peeled and diced

3 stalks celery, diced

½ cup sliced white mushrooms

½ cup chopped spinach

2 cups cauliflower rice

1½ pounds ground pork

2 tablespoons coconut aminos

1 teaspoon salt

½ teaspoon freshly ground black pepper

½ teaspoon ground sage

¼ teaspoon chopped fresh parsley

1½ cups shredded mozzarella cheese

1. Heat olive oil in a medium skillet over medium heat. Add garlic and cook until fragrant, about 2 minutes. Add onion and celery and cook until softened, about 4 minutes. Add mushrooms and spinach and cook until mushrooms are softened and spinach is wilted, another 4 minutes.

2. Add cauliflower rice and cook until softened but still slightly crisp, about 2 minutes. Add pork, coconut aminos, salt, pepper, sage, and parsley and cook until pork is no longer pink, about 7 minutes.

3. Sprinkle cheese on top and cover; cook until cheese is melted, about 5 minutes.

4. Allow to cool slightly, then divide into six equal portions and place each portion in an airtight container. Store in the refrigerator until ready to eat.

PER SERVING Calories: 389 | Fat: 30 g | Protein: 20 g | Sodium: 634 mg | Fiber: 2 g | Carbohydrates: 7 g | Sugar: 3 g

Pork and Red Peppers

When preparing your menu for the week, note which recipes require you to marinate meat. Quickly prepare the marinades the night before you want to cook and let the meat sit in them overnight in the refrigerator to save time on the day of cooking. This finished dish will keep in the refrigerator up to 1 week.

INGREDIENTS | SERVES 6

3 cloves garlic, minced

1 teaspoon salt

1 teaspoon freshly ground black pepper

2 tablespoons olive oil, divided

1½ pounds pork tenderloin, cut into 1" medallions

¼ cup chopped red onion

2 medium red bell peppers, seeded and cut into thin slices

1 cup no-sugar-added chicken broth

1 teaspoon arrowroot powder

2 teaspoons water

1 tablespoon lemon juice

Chicken Broth versus Bone Broth

The main difference between chicken broth and bone broth is the amount of time the broths are allowed to simmer. Both are typically made with chicken bones, but unlike chicken broth, which simmers for about an hour, bone broth simmers for 4–24 hours. The long simmering time helps extract important nutrients like amino acids and collagen from the bones. If you want to up the nutritional value of any of your recipes, you can replace chicken broth with bone broth.

1. Combine garlic, salt, pepper, and 1 tablespoon olive oil in a large bowl and stir to mix well. Add pork slices to bowl, toss to coat, cover, and allow to sit in the refrigerator 2 hours or overnight.

2. Heat remaining olive oil in a large skillet over high heat. Add pork and garlic mixture and sear pork 1 minute on each side to brown. Remove pork from skillet.

3. Reduce heat to medium and add onions and peppers to skillet. Cook until slightly softened, about 3 minutes. Pour in chicken broth and use a wooden spoon to scrape the bottom of the pan.

4. Combine arrowroot powder and water, stir to mix well, and stir mixture into chicken broth. Allow to cook 2 minutes or until slightly thickened.

5. Add pork back to skillet and cook 12 minutes or until pork is fully cooked through, turning once while cooking.

6. Pour lemon juice over pork slices and remove from heat.

7. Divide into six equal portions and transfer each portion to an airtight container. Store in the refrigerator.

PER SERVING   Calories: 186 | Fat: 7 g | Protein: 24 g | Sodium: 461 mg | Fiber: 1 g | Carbohydrates: 4 g | Sugar: 2 g

Ground Pork Chili

The flavors in this chili lend themselves well to any ground meat—beef, chicken, turkey, or pork. If any of the other ground meats are more to your liking, you can substitute one or a combination for the pork. This chili will last in the refrigerator up to 1 week.

INGREDIENTS | SERVES 6

2 tablespoons olive oil, divided

1½ pounds ground pork

2 teaspoons salt, divided

½ teaspoon freshly ground black pepper

3 cloves garlic, minced

1 large yellow onion, peeled and diced

2 medium green bell peppers, seeded and diced

1 medium red bell pepper, seeded and diced

1 tablespoon minced pickled jalapeño

1 (14.5-ounce) can diced fire-roasted tomatoes

1 (15-ounce) can no-sugar-added tomato sauce

1 (4-ounce) can tomato paste

1 tablespoon chili powder

½ teaspoon dried marjoram

½ teaspoon dried oregano

¼ teaspoon ground nutmeg

1. Heat 1 tablespoon olive oil in a stockpot over medium heat. Add pork, 1 teaspoon salt, and pepper and cook until pork is no longer pink, about 7 minutes. Scoop pork from pot with a slotted spoon and set aside.

2. Add remaining olive oil to pot and stir in garlic and onions. Cook until softened, about 4 minutes. Add diced peppers and jalapeños and cook until peppers start to soften, another 4 minutes.

3. Return pork to pot along with remaining ingredients and stir to mix well. Reduce heat to low and simmer for 1 hour.

4. Remove from heat and divide into six equal portions. Store each portion in a separate airtight container in the refrigerator until ready to eat.

PER SERVING Calories: 404 | Fat: 28 g | Protein: 22 g | Sodium: 1,222 mg | Fiber: 5 g | Carbohydrates: 14 g | Sugar: 8 g

Italian Pork Soup

This soup freezes and reheats very well. If you want to freeze it for later, measure out portions and put each portion in its own freezer-safe container. When you're ready to eat it, you can take one portion out at a time to thaw. This will last in the freezer up to 3 months or up to 1 week in the refrigerator.

INGREDIENTS | SERVES 6

1 tablespoon olive oil

3 cloves garlic, minced

1 medium yellow onion, peeled and chopped

1 cup chopped red bell pepper

½ cup sliced white mushrooms

1½ pounds pork chops, cut into 1" cubes

1 (14-ounce) can quartered artichoke hearts, roughly chopped

¼ cup chopped sun-dried tomatoes

1 (14.5-ounce) can fire-roasted tomatoes

1 quart no-sugar-added chicken broth

1 tablespoon Italian seasoning

1 teaspoon salt

½ teaspoon freshly ground black pepper

1 cup chopped spinach

1. Heat olive oil in a stockpot over medium heat. Add garlic and onions and cook until softened, about 4 minutes. Add bell pepper and mushrooms and cook until softened but still slightly crisp, about 4 minutes.

2. Add pork chops and cook until no longer pink, about 8 minutes.

3. Add all remaining ingredients except spinach to pot and bring to a boil. Reduce heat to low and simmer 30 minutes. Remove from heat and stir in spinach.

4. Allow to cool and then divide into six equal portions and transfer each portion to a separate airtight container. Store in the refrigerator until ready to eat.

PER SERVING   Calories: 229 | Fat: 8 g | Protein: 29 g | Sodium: 591 mg | Fiber: 3 g | Carbohydrates: 10 g | Sugar: 5 g

What Are Fire-Roasted Tomatoes?

Fire-roasted tomatoes have been picked at their peak flavor, roasted over an open fire until charred and crisp on the outside, and then diced and canned. Using fire-roasted tomatoes adds a smoky, chargrilled flavor to any dish, but if you prefer the taste of raw tomatoes, you can substitute regular or petite diced tomatoes in any recipe that calls for fire-roasted.

Sausage Jalapeño Poppers

These little gems are divine warm or cold. You can eat them right out of the refrigerator, but if you want to heat them up, broil them in the oven 2–3 minutes or until cheese is bubbly again. They will keep up to 1 week in the refrigerator, if they last that long!

INGREDIENTS | SERVES 6 (2 HALVES PER SERVING)

½ pound ground no-sugar-added pork sausage

4 ounces cream cheese, softened

½ cup shredded Asiago cheese

6 large jalapeños, cut in half lengthwise and seeded

1. Preheat oven to 350°F.

2. Crumble sausage into a small skillet over medium heat and cook until no longer pink, about 7 minutes. Transfer sausage to a paper towel–lined plate.

3. Combine sausage, cream cheese, and Asiago cheese in a medium bowl and stir to mix well.

4. Spoon about 1 tablespoon of mixture into each jalapeño half and arrange jalapeños on a baking sheet.

5. Bake 30 minutes or until bubbly and slightly browned.

6. Transfer two halves to each of six airtight containers and store in the refrigerator until ready to eat.

PER SERVING Calories: 249 | Fat: 21 g | Protein: 12 g | Sodium: 272 mg | Fiber: 0 g | Carbohydrates: 1 g | Sugar: 0 g

Pork Ragu

You can create a low-carb dish similar to traditional ragu by scooping some of this Pork Ragu onto ½ cup cooked spaghetti squash or zucchini noodles. This dish will last up to 1 week in the refrigerator.

INGREDIENTS | SERVES 6

2 teaspoons dried rosemary

1 teaspoon salt

1 teaspoon freshly ground black pepper

1½ pounds pork shoulder, cut into 1" cubes

2 tablespoons olive oil

1 tablespoon ghee

2 cloves garlic, minced

1 medium yellow onion, peeled and diced

2 tablespoons tomato paste

1½ cups no-sugar-added chicken broth

2 (14.5-ounce) cans petite diced tomatoes

What Is Ragu?

Traditionally, ragu is a meat-based Italian sauce that's made with ground meat, onions, tomatoes, and red wine and served with pasta. It was created in Italy in the eighteenth century by a man named Alberto Alvisi. This low-carb ragu has all the flavors of the real thing but swaps out some ingredients to keep the carbohydrate count lower.

1. Combine herbs and spices in a large bowl and stir to mix well. Add pork to bowl and toss to coat.

2. Heat olive oil and ghee in a medium skillet over medium heat. Add garlic and cook until fragrant, about 2 minutes. Add onions and continue cooking until softened, about 4 minutes. Stir tomato paste into pan and add pork. Cook until pork is browned on all sides, about 10 minutes.

3. Stir in ½ cup chicken broth and scrape the bottom of the pan with a wooden spoon to release any browned bits. Add remaining chicken broth and diced tomatoes and allow to simmer 30 minutes or until pork is fully cooked and sauce is thickened.

4. Remove from heat and divide into six equal portions. Store each portion in a separate airtight container and refrigerate until ready to eat.

PER SERVING   Calories: 272 | Fat: 15 g | Protein: 24 g | Sodium: 542 mg | Fiber: 2 g | Carbohydrates: 9 g | Sugar: 5 g

Sausage Casserole

For an easier way to take this casserole on the go, pour prepared egg mixture into greased muffin tins and bake 30 minutes or until set. If you do it this way, you can store individual "muffins" in your freezer up to 3 months until you're ready to eat them. Or make the dish as instructed and store it in the refrigerator up to 1 week.

INGREDIENTS | SERVES 6

½ pound ground no-sugar-added pork sausage

8 large eggs, beaten

1 cup cottage cheese

½ cup shredded Cheddar cheese

1 (4-ounce) can green chilies

½ teaspoon salt

½ teaspoon freshly ground black pepper

1 tablespoon butter

2 tablespoons minced green onion

¼ cup sliced white mushrooms

1. Preheat oven to 350°F.

2. Cook sausage in a small skillet over medium heat until no longer brown, about 7 minutes. Transfer sausage to a plate lined with a paper towel to absorb excess grease.

3. Combine eggs, cottage cheese, Cheddar cheese, green chilies, salt, and pepper in a medium bowl and stir to mix well. Set aside.

4. Heat butter in the same skillet over medium heat. Add green onions and mushrooms and cook until mushrooms are softened, about 4 minutes. Allow to cool and then add onion, mushrooms, and cooked sausage to egg mixture and stir to incorporate.

5. Pour into a greased 9" × 13" pan and bake 45 minutes or until set. Remove from oven and allow to cool.

6. Cut into six equal servings and transfer each serving to a separate airtight container. Store in the refrigerator until ready to eat.

PER SERVING Calories: 393 | Fat: 31 g | Protein: 23 g | Sodium: 534 mg | Fiber: 1 g | Carbohydrates: 5 g | Sugar: 2 g

Pork Chop Stew

You can make a quicker version of this stew by adding some cooked Easy Shredded Chicken (Chapter 13) from your pressure cooker instead of pork and skipping the first hour of simmering. Better yet, make a batch of each and freeze some for later. This stew will keep up to 1 week in the refrigerator.

INGREDIENTS | SERVES 6

12 ounces bone-in pork chops

1 teaspoon garlic powder

1 teaspoon paprika

½ teaspoon chili powder

½ teaspoon dried oregano

1 teaspoon salt

½ teaspoon freshly ground black pepper

1 bay leaf

4 cups no-sugar-added chicken broth

2 tablespoons coconut aminos

1½ cups peeled and cubed turnips

1 cup chopped bok choy

½ cup chopped carrots

1 medium yellow onion, peeled and diced

2 stalks celery, diced

1. Combine pork chops, garlic powder, paprika, chili powder, oregano, salt, pepper, bay leaf, chicken broth, and coconut aminos in a large stockpot. Bring to a boil over high heat, reduce heat to medium low, and simmer 1 hour.

2. Remove pork chops and allow to cool. Cut into bite-sized pieces and discard bones. Return cut pieces to pot.

3. Add remaining ingredients, stir to combine, and bring to a boil over high heat. Reduce heat to medium low and simmer 1 more hour. Remove bay leaf.

4. Divide into six equal portions and put each portion into a separate airtight container. Store in the refrigerator until ready to eat.

PER SERVING   Calories: 168 | Fat: 8 g | Protein: 15 g | Sodium: 680 mg | Fiber: 2 g | Carbohydrates: 9 g | Sugar: 3 g

Curry Pork Burgers

If you prefer to make these pork burgers on the stove, heat coconut oil over medium-high heat and cook burgers in a medium skillet 5 minutes on each side or until pork is no longer pink. These burgers will keep up to 1 week in the refrigerator.

INGREDIENTS | SERVES 6

2 tablespoons coconut oil

1½ pounds ground pork

¾ cup crumbled feta cheese

¾ cup chopped fresh parsley

3 tablespoons yellow curry paste

3 cloves garlic, minced

1 teaspoon Worcestershire sauce

2 scallions, green parts only, chopped

1 tablespoon minced dried onion

½ teaspoon dried ginger

1 teaspoon ground cumin

½ teaspoon salt

¼ teaspoon freshly ground black pepper

1. Preheat grill to medium-high heat and oil grate with coconut oil.

2. Combine all remaining ingredients in a medium bowl and mix well to incorporate. Divide into six equal portions and shape each portion into a patty.

3. Place burgers on grill and cook until pork is cooked through, about 5 minutes on each side. Remove from grill and allow to cool.

4. Transfer each patty to a separate airtight container and store in the refrigerator until ready to eat.

PER SERVING Calories: 393 | Fat: 32 g | Protein: 22 g | Sodium: 443 mg | Fiber: 0 g | Carbohydrates: 2 g | Sugar: 1 g

What Is Curry Paste?

Although there are different variations, curry paste is a combination of chilies, garlic, lemongrass, ginger, curry, coriander, turmeric, and cumin. These ingredients are blended together to form a flavorful paste with a texture similar to lumpy mayonnaise. Curry paste comes in yellow or red and can be found in the international section of your grocery store.

CHAPTER 7

Vegetarian and Vegan

Chai Chia Pudding

If you don't have glass Mason jars, you can store this pudding in any airtight containers. It will last in the refrigerator up to 1 week and will thicken as the week goes on. You can eat it thick or add a little coconut milk or water right before eating to thin it out a little bit.

INGREDIENTS | SERVES 6

4 cups brewed chai tea
¾ cup chia seeds
1 teaspoon vanilla extract
1 cup full-fat coconut milk
5 drops liquid stevia

Making Your Own Chai

If you don't have chai tea handy to brew, you can replace the chai tea with coconut or almond milk and add 1½ teaspoons ground cinnamon, 1 teaspoon ground ginger, ½ teaspoon ground cardamom, and ⅛ teaspoon ground cloves.

1. Combine all ingredients in a blender. Blend until smooth.

2. Pour equal amounts of mixture into six separate glass Mason jars. Cover and allow to set in the refrigerator at least 2 hours.

3. Store in the refrigerator until ready to eat.

PER SERVING   Calories: 147 | Fat: 13 g | Protein: 4 g | Sodium: 10 mg | Fiber: 4.5 g | Carbohydrates: 6 g | Sugar: 0 g

Vegetarian Pancakes

These vegetarian pancakes come together in less than 10 minutes. If you prefer a savory flavor, leave out the cinnamon and vanilla, and they can be used as a sandwich wrap. These pancakes will keep up to 1 week in the refrigerator.

INGREDIENTS | SERVES 6 (2 PANCAKES PER SERVING)

1 tablespoon butter, softened
6 ounces cream cheese, softened
6 large eggs
½ teaspoon ground cinnamon
½ teaspoon vanilla extract
1 tablespoon coconut oil

1. Combine all ingredients except coconut oil in a blender and process until smooth.

2. Heat coconut oil in a medium skillet over medium heat. Pour batter onto hot skillet by ¼ cupfuls. Cook each pancake 2 minutes and then flip and cook 2 more minutes or until golden brown.

3. Transfer two pancakes to each of six airtight containers and store in the refrigerator until ready to eat.

PER SERVING   Calories: 205 | Fat: 18 g | Protein: 8 g | Sodium: 173 mg | Fiber: 0 g | Carbohydrates: 1 g | Sugar: 1 g

Cauliflower Fried Rice

Traditional fried rice uses carrots and edamame, but this version is both low-carb and soy-free. If you want to make it vegan, just leave out the eggs and swap the ghee for olive or coconut oil. This fried rice will last up to 1 week in the refrigerator.

INGREDIENTS | SERVES 6

3 tablespoons ghee, divided

2 large eggs, lightly beaten

½ cup diced yellow onion

3 cloves garlic, minced

2 stalks celery, diced

3 cups riced cauliflower

4 tablespoons coconut aminos

¼ teaspoon salt

¼ teaspoon crushed red pepper flakes

2 tablespoons sesame oil

3 tablespoons minced scallions, green parts only

¼ cup chopped cashews

1. Heat 1 tablespoon ghee in a medium skillet over medium-low heat. Add eggs to pan and scramble until cooked through, about 4 minutes. Remove from skillet and set aside.

2. In the same skillet, heat remaining ghee over medium-high heat. Add onions and cook until softened, about 4 minutes. Add garlic and cook 1 more minute. Add celery and cook 3 more minutes.

3. Add cauliflower, coconut aminos, salt, and red pepper flakes to pan. Cook until cauliflower is softened, about 4 minutes.

4. Remove from heat and stir in scrambled eggs, sesame oil, scallions, and cashews.

5. Divide into six equal portions and store each portion in a separate airtight container. Store in the refrigerator until ready to eat.

PER SERVING Calories: 180 | Fat: 14 g | Protein: 5 g | Sodium: 444 mg | Fiber: 2 g | Carbohydrates: 8 g | Sugar: 3 g

Chow Mein Zoodles

If you prefer a crispier "noodle," don't add zucchini noodles to the pan while cooking. Leave them out and pour prepared vegetables and sauce over noodles while they're still hot, tossing to coat. This will soften the noodles without the extra cooking time. This dish will keep up to 1 week in the refrigerator.

INGREDIENTS | SERVES 6

½ cup coconut aminos

1½ teaspoons granulated erythritol

1½ tablespoons arrowroot powder

3 teaspoons sesame oil

¼ teaspoon freshly ground black pepper

1 teaspoon crushed red pepper flakes

2 tablespoons water

2 tablespoons olive oil

3 cloves garlic, minced

½ teaspoon minced fresh ginger

1½ cups shredded green cabbage

1 cup broccoli florets, cut into bite-sized pieces

3 cups zucchini noodles

2 tablespoons sesame seeds

Chow Mein versus Lo Mein

Chow mein and lo mein are similar dishes, yet they have one distinct difference. Although the ingredients are typically the same (or very similar), chow mein involves panfrying noodles to give them a crispy texture, whereas lo mein calls for boiling noodles to give them a soft texture.

1. Combine coconut aminos, erythritol, arrowroot powder, sesame oil, black pepper, red pepper flakes, and water in a small bowl and whisk to combine. Set aside.

2. Heat olive oil in a large skillet over medium-high heat. Add garlic and ginger; cook until fragrant, about 2 minutes. Add cabbage and cook 2–3 minutes until softened but still slightly crisp. Add broccoli and cook until softened but still slightly crisp, about 3 minutes. Add zucchini noodles to the skillet and cook 2 minutes. Pour in sauce, toss to coat, and remove from heat.

3. Sprinkle sesame seeds over mixture and toss to coat.

4. Divide into six equal portions and store each portion in a separate airtight container. Store in the refrigerator until ready to eat.

PER SERVING Calories: 126 | Fat: 8 g | Protein: 4 g | Sodium: 592 mg | Fiber: 2 g | Carbohydrates: 11 g | Sugar: 3 g

Broccoli Cheese Veggie Balls

These balls make a perfect nutrient-packed snack or side. You can also add a poached egg or two on the top before eating them for a vegetable-rich breakfast that's ready to go in minutes. They will last up to 1 week in the refrigerator.

INGREDIENTS | SERVES 6 (4 BALLS PER SERVING)

½ cup water
4 cups broccoli florets
½ cup coarsely ground almond meal
¾ cup Parmesan cheese
¼ cup shredded Cheddar cheese
2 cloves garlic, minced
1 teaspoon salt
½ teaspoon freshly ground black pepper
½ teaspoon dried parsley
1 large egg, beaten

Making Your Own Almond Meal

If you want to make your own almond meal, put 1 cup of almonds in a food processor and pulse until you get a coarse meal. Make sure not to overprocess. You want the almond meal to have a grainy texture similar to a thick sand.

1. Preheat oven to 350°F.

2. Combine water and broccoli florets in a medium saucepan and turn to medium-high heat. Allow to steam 8 minutes or until broccoli is softened.

3. Pour excess water out of pan and mash broccoli using a potato masher. Add remaining ingredients and stir to combine.

4. Shape mixture into twenty-four equal-sized balls and arrange balls on a baking sheet lined with parchment paper.

5. Bake 20 minutes or until balls turn golden brown. Remove from oven and allow to cool.

6. Transfer four cooked veggie balls to each of six separate airtight containers and store in the refrigerator until ready to eat.

PER SERVING Calories: 115 | Fat: 8 g | Protein: 7 g | Sodium: 472 mg | Fiber: 3 g | Carbohydrates: 7 g | Sugar: 1 g

Spaghetti Squash Lasagna

If you have cooked spaghetti squash and jarred marinara sauce on hand, this recipe comes together in no time. You can make two lasagnas, cook one, and put the other one in the freezer until you're ready to cook it. This cooked lasagna lasts up to 1 week in the refrigerator.

INGREDIENTS | SERVES 6

1 large egg
1½ cups cottage cheese
½ cup ricotta cheese
¼ cup grated Parmesan cheese
3 tablespoons minced fresh parsley
3 cups baby spinach, chopped
2¼ cups no-sugar-added marinara sauce
4 cups cooked spaghetti squash
4 slices provolone cheese
1 cup shredded mozzarella cheese

1. Preheat oven to 350°F.

2. Beat egg in a medium mixing bowl. Add cottage cheese, ricotta cheese, and Parmesan cheese and stir to combine. Stir in parsley and spinach. Set aside.

3. Pour ¾ cup marinara sauce into the bottom of a 9" × 9" baking dish and spread evenly. Add 2 cups spaghetti squash on top and spread evenly. Top with half the cottage cheese mixture. Add provolone slices in a single layer.

4. Pour ¾ cup marinara sauce over provolone slices, add remaining spaghetti squash on top of that, and then spread remaining cottage cheese mixture on top. Pour remaining sauce on top of cottage cheese mixture and spread evenly. Sprinkle with mozzarella cheese.

5. Bake uncovered 40 minutes or until hot and bubbling with cheese starting to brown. Remove from oven and allow to cool.

6. Cut into six equal portions and transfer each portion to a separate airtight container. Store in the refrigerator until ready to eat.

PER SERVING Calories: 332 | Fat: 18 g | Protein: 21 g | Sodium: 918 mg | Fiber: 5 g | Carbohydrates: 22 g | Sugar: 10 g

Spicy Cauliflower Burgers

You can eat these burgers as is or turn them into wraps by chopping up the cooked burger and placing the chopped pieces into one of the Vegetarian Pancakes cooked savory style (see recipe in this chapter) and adding your favorite toppings. These patties will last up to 1 week in the refrigerator.

INGREDIENTS | SERVES 6

2 tablespoons olive oil

2 cloves garlic, minced

1 cup chopped yellow onion

½ cup chopped spinach

8 ounces baby bella mushrooms, chopped

2 cups grated cauliflower

1 tablespoon coconut aminos

1 teaspoon cumin

½ teaspoon chili powder

⅛ teaspoon ground cayenne pepper

¼ cup unblanched almond flour

Grating Your Cauliflower

You can grate cauliflower two ways: with a cheese grater or a food processor. If you're using a handheld cheese grater, cut cauliflower head into large pieces and slowly and carefully grate until you have the desired quantity. If you're using a food processor, put grating attachment in place and add cauliflower, using care not to overprocess.

1. Preheat oven to 400°F.

2. Heat olive oil in a medium skillet over medium heat. Add garlic and cook until fragrant, about 2 minutes. Add onion, spinach, and mushrooms and cook until softened, about 4 minutes.

3. Add all remaining ingredients except almond flour and cook until cauliflower starts to soften, about 3 minutes.

4. Remove from heat and allow to cool. Stir in almond flour.

5. Divide mixture into six equal portions and shape into patties. Line patties in a single layer on a baking sheet lined with parchment paper.

6. Bake 30 minutes, carefully turning once while cooking. Remove from oven and allow to cool.

7. Transfer each patty to a separate airtight container and store in the refrigerator until ready to eat.

PER SERVING Calories: 100 | Fat: 7 g | Protein: 4 g | Sodium: 95 mg | Fiber: 2 g | Carbohydrates: 7 g | Sugar: 3 g

Basil Soup

This soup may thicken a little bit as it sits in the refrigerator. If you want to thin it out a little, stir in a little bit of vegetable broth right before reheating. You can keep this soup in your refrigerator up to 1 week.

INGREDIENTS | SERVES 6

2 tablespoons avocado oil

3 tablespoons minced garlic

1 large white onion, peeled and diced

6 large zucchini, diced

1 cup packed fresh basil

4 cups vegetable broth

1 teaspoon salt

1 teaspoon freshly ground black pepper

½ teaspoon crushed red pepper flakes

½ cup full-fat coconut milk

1. Heat avocado oil in a large saucepan over medium heat. Add garlic and cook until fragrant, about 2 minutes. Add onion and continue cooking until softened, about 4 minutes.

2. Add zucchini and cook until slightly softened but still crisp, about 3 minutes.

3. Add remaining ingredients except coconut milk and stir to combine. Bring soup to a boil and then reduce heat to low and allow to simmer 5 minutes or until zucchini is softened.

4. Use an immersion blender to blend soup into a purée. If you don't have an immersion blender, transfer contents to a blender and blend until smooth. Stir in coconut milk.

5. Divide into six equal portions and store each portion in a separate airtight container in the refrigerator until ready to eat.

PER SERVING Calories: 151 | Fat: 9 g | Protein: 5 g | Sodium: 517 mg | Fiber: 4 g | Carbohydrates: 14 g | Sugar: 9 g

Grilled Cauliflower with Sesame Sauce

If you prefer to cook in your oven, set it to 400°F and roast cauliflower for 20–25 minutes or until crispy and golden brown, rotating every 5 minutes. This dish will keep up to 1 week in the refrigerator.

INGREDIENTS | SERVES 6

1 large cauliflower head, cut in large florets

2 tablespoons olive oil

1 teaspoon garlic powder

1 teaspoon onion powder

¼ teaspoon ground ginger

4 tablespoons coconut aminos

4 tablespoons tahini

1 teaspoon red chili paste

2 tablespoons sesame seeds

1. Combine cauliflower and olive oil in a medium bowl and toss to coat. Sprinkle garlic powder, onion powder, and ginger on top and toss again.

2. Heat grill to medium heat and cook cauliflower until golden brown, about 12 minutes, rotating every 2 minutes to prevent it from burning. Remove cauliflower from grill and set aside.

3. Whisk together coconut aminos, tahini, and chili paste in a medium bowl. Add cauliflower to bowl and toss to coat completely. Sprinkle on sesame seeds and toss to incorporate.

4. Divide cauliflower into six equal portions and store each portion in a separate airtight container in the refrigerator until ready to eat.

PER SERVING Calories: 163 | Fat: 12 g | Protein: 6 g | Sodium: 343 mg | Fiber: 4 g | Carbohydrates: 12 g | Sugar: 3 g

Tomato Basil Zoodles

This recipe doesn't require you to cook the zucchini noodles. If you want them cooked, you can sauté them with a little olive oil for 2–3 minutes. Separate the sauce from the cooked zucchini while storing in the refrigerator and then combine them right before you're ready to eat. This dish will keep up to 1 week in the refrigerator.

INGREDIENTS | SERVES 6

1 cup fresh basil

1 clove garlic

⅛ cup pine nuts

⅓ cup plus 1 tablespoon olive oil, divided

½ teaspoon salt

¼ teaspoon freshly ground black pepper

⅓ cup chopped yellow onion

1 cup cherry tomatoes, quartered

⅓ cup crushed walnuts

3 large zucchini, spiralized

The Power of Pine Nuts

Pine nuts don't get as much attention as almonds, but they should become a regular part of your low-carb diet. These little nuts contain fatty acids that trigger your body to release cholecystokinin, or CCK—a hormone that helps suppress your appetite. Pine nuts are also a good source of magnesium, which fights fatigue, and monounsaturated fat, iron, and protein—three nutrients that also boost energy.

1. Combine basil, garlic, and pine nuts in a food processor and pulse until coarsely chopped. With food processor running, slowly pour in ⅓ cup olive oil until pesto is smooth. Add salt and pepper and pulse once or twice to incorporate.

2. Add remaining olive oil to a medium skillet and set to medium heat. Add onions and cook until softened, about 4 minutes. Add tomatoes and cook until softened, about 4 more minutes. Add walnuts and prepared pesto sauce and cook 2 more minutes.

3. Allow sauce mixture to cool slightly and then toss with zucchini noodles. Divide into six equal portions and store each portion in a separate airtight container. Store in the refrigerator until ready to eat.

PER SERVING Calories: 189 | Fat: 17 g | Protein: 4 g | Sodium: 209 mg | Fiber: 3 g | Carbohydrates: 8 g | Sugar: 5 g

Cauliflower Mac 'n' Cheese

With this low-carb recipe, missing macaroni and cheese has become a thing of the past. If you want a more traditional pasta feel, you can replace the cauliflower with cooked spaghetti squash. You can keep this dish up to 1 week in the refrigerator.

INGREDIENTS | SERVES 6

2 tablespoons olive oil

1 teaspoon salt

½ teaspoon freshly ground black pepper

¼ teaspoon granulated garlic

1 teaspoon dried parsley

1 large head cauliflower, cut into bite-sized florets

1 cup shredded Cheddar cheese

½ cup shredded Gruyère cheese

½ cup full-fat coconut milk

1 tablespoon ghee

⅛ teaspoon ground nutmeg

¼ cup grated Parmesan cheese

Veganize It

If you want to make a vegan version of this recipe, you can make a vegan cheese sauce by combining 1 (15-ounce) can full-fat coconut milk, 2 tablespoons no-sugar-added cashew butter, 1 tablespoon olive oil, 1 teaspoon onion powder, ½ teaspoon garlic powder, ¾ teaspoon dry mustard, ½ teaspoon salt, ½ teaspoon pepper, 5 tablespoons nutritional yeast, and ½ teaspoon white vinegar in a food processor and processing until smooth. Heat sauce over low heat on the stove and pour on top of cauliflower before baking.

1. Preheat oven to 450°F. Line a baking sheet with parchment paper.

2. In a medium mixing bowl, combine olive oil, salt, pepper, garlic, and parsley. Add cauliflower and toss to coat.

3. Arrange cauliflower on a baking sheet in a single layer. Roast 15 minutes or until browned and crispy. Transfer cauliflower to an 8" × 8" baking dish.

4. Combine remaining ingredients except Parmesan cheese in a medium saucepan over medium heat. Stir and allow to simmer 5 minutes. Pour over cauliflower and toss to coat completely. Sprinkle Parmesan cheese on top.

5. Bake 10 minutes or until starting to brown. Remove and allow to cool.

6. Divide into six equal portions and transfer each portion to an airtight container. Store in the refrigerator until ready to eat.

PER SERVING   Calories: 273 | Fat: 23 g | Protein: 12 g | Sodium: 715 mg | Fiber: 2 g | Carbohydrates: 6 g | Sugar: 2 g

Pan-Fried Eggplant

Don't skip the first step of this recipe. Letting the sliced eggplant sit with the salt before cooking draws excess moisture out. This gives you a crispier eggplant, which is ideal, especially when storing the eggplant for a few days before you eat it. This will keep for up to 1 week in the refrigerator.

INGREDIENTS | SERVES 6

1 large eggplant, cut into ¼" slices

2 teaspoons salt, divided

½ cup full-fat coconut milk

1 cup almond flour

1 tablespoon dried parsley

2 teaspoons granulated garlic

1 teaspoon granulated onion

½ teaspoon freshly ground black pepper

½ cup coconut oil

1. Arrange eggplant slices in a single layer on a baking sheet lined with paper towels. Sprinkle 1 teaspoon salt over slices and let sit 30 minutes. After 30 minutes, blot excess moisture from eggplant with a paper towel.

2. Pour coconut milk into a small bowl. In a separate medium bowl, combine all remaining ingredients except coconut oil and eggplant.

3. Dip each slice of eggplant into coconut milk and then coat in almond flour mixture.

4. Heat coconut oil in a medium skillet over medium-high heat. Drop coated eggplant slices in a single layer into hot oil. Cook 3 minutes then flip over and cook 3–4 minutes or until browned and crispy.

5. Transfer cooked eggplant to a plate lined with a paper towel to absorb excess oil.

6. After excess oil is absorbed, divide slices into six equal portions and transfer to an airtight container. Store in the refrigerator until ready to eat.

PER SERVING Calories: 300 | Fat: 22 g | Protein: 4 g | Sodium: 469 mg | Fiber: 3 g | Carbohydrates: 10 g | Sugar: 3 g

Spinach Pie

If you want to make this recipe more portable, you can pour the mixture directly into greased muffin tins and cook it that way. You can keep this in the refrigerator up to 1 week.

INGREDIENTS | SERVES 6

2 tablespoons olive oil

1 medium yellow onion, peeled and chopped

1 (16-ounce) package frozen chopped spinach, thawed and drained

¼ cup chopped scallions

⅛ teaspoon ground nutmeg

1 teaspoon garlic salt

6 large eggs, beaten

2 cups shredded Muenster cheese

1 cup shredded Swiss cheese

1. Preheat oven to 350°F. Lightly grease a 9" pie plate.

2. Heat olive oil in a skillet over medium heat. Add onion and cook until softened, about 4 minutes. Add spinach and cook until heated through, about 3 more minutes.

3. Combine remaining ingredients in a medium bowl. Add spinach mixture and stir to mix well.

4. Pour prepared mixture into pie plate and bake 30 minutes or until eggs have set.

5. Cut into six equal portions and transfer each portion to a separate airtight container. Store in the refrigerator until ready to eat.

PER SERVING Calories: 399 | Fat: 30 g | Protein: 25 g | Sodium: 817 mg | Fiber: 2 g | Carbohydrates: 7 g | Sugar: 2 g

Turnip Fries

These fries will soften as they're stored in the refrigerator, but they are still delicious that way. If you want to crisp them up, broil them 3–4 minutes right before eating, flipping once while broiling. They will keep up to 1 week in the refrigerator.

INGREDIENTS | SERVES 6

6 medium turnips, peeled and cut into 2" vertical sticks

2 tablespoons avocado oil

1 teaspoon salt

½ teaspoon freshly ground black pepper

½ teaspoon paprika

1. Preheat oven to 425°F.

2. Combine all ingredients in a medium bowl and toss to coat.

3. Spread coated turnip sticks out in a single layer on a baking sheet lined with parchment paper.

4. Roast 25 minutes, flipping once during cooking.

5. Divide into six equal portions and store in an airtight container until ready to eat.

PER SERVING Calories: 74 | Fat: 5 g | Protein: 1 g | Sodium: 469 mg | Fiber: 2 g | Carbohydrates: 8 g | Sugar: 5 g

Mushroom Burgers

For a complete vegetarian meal, pair these mushroom burgers with a side of Turnip Fries (see recipe in this chapter), Zucchini Tots (Chapter 10), or Cheesy Cauliflower Tots (Chapter 10), and a dollop of homemade Ketchup (Chapter 9). These burgers will keep in the refrigerator up to 1 week.

INGREDIENTS | SERVES 6

1 pound baby bella mushrooms

1 large yellow onion, peeled and roughly chopped

2 tablespoons coconut aminos

1 large egg

1 teaspoon salt

1 teaspoon freshly ground black pepper

½ teaspoon granulated onion

½ teaspoon granulated garlic

3 tablespoons olive oil

1. Combine all ingredients except olive oil in a food processor and pulse until combined but not puréed. The goal is to create a meat-like texture.

2. Form mixture into six equal-sized patties.

3. Heat olive oil in a medium skillet over medium-high heat and cook 3–4 minutes on each side or until crispy and slightly browned.

4. Transfer each mushroom burger to an airtight container and store in the refrigerator until ready to eat.

PER SERVING Calories: 105 | Fat: 7 g | Protein: 4 g | Sodium: 549 mg | Fiber: 1 g | Carbohydrates: 6 g | Sugar: 3 g

Thai Chopped Salad

Storing the salad dressing in a separate container until you're ready to eat the salad ensures that the vegetables will stay crunchy. This salad will last in the refrigerator up to 1 week.

INGREDIENTS | SERVES 6

1 (15-ounce) can full-fat coconut milk

¼ cup no-sugar-added almond butter

1 tablespoon curry powder

⅛ teaspoon cayenne pepper

2 cloves garlic

2 tablespoons lime juice

1 teaspoon salt

3 cups baby kale

2 cups chopped green cabbage

1 medium red bell pepper, seeded and chopped

1 medium yellow bell pepper, seeded and chopped

½ cup chopped cilantro

½ cup chopped almonds

1. Combine coconut milk, almond butter, curry powder, cayenne pepper, garlic, lime juice, and salt in a blender or food processor and process until smooth. Divide into six equal portions and transfer each portion to a small airtight container.

2. Combine remaining ingredients in a medium bowl and toss to incorporate. Divide into six equal portions and transfer each portion to an airtight container. Store a container of dressing in each salad container and refrigerate until ready to eat.

PER SERVING Calories: 298 | Fat: 26 g | Protein: 8 g | Sodium: 453 mg | Fiber: 4 g | Carbohydrates: 12 g | Sugar: 4 g

Spinach and Artichoke Spaghetti Squash

This recipe calls for cooked spaghetti squash, which is nice to have on hand at all times when meal prepping for a low-carb diet. You can use the pressure cooker method or the oven method (see sidebar) to cook your spaghetti squash. This cooked dish will keep in the refrigerator up to 1 week.

INGREDIENTS | SERVES 6

1 tablespoon olive oil

3 cloves garlic, minced

½ cup chopped yellow onion

½ cup sliced white mushrooms

½ cup Basic Mayonnaise (Chapter 9)

3 ounces cream cheese

1 teaspoon salt

½ teaspoon freshly ground black pepper

⅛ teaspoon ground nutmeg

½ cup shredded Parmesan cheese

3 cups baby spinach

1 (14-ounce) can artichoke hearts

3 cups cooked spaghetti squash

½ cup shredded mozzarella cheese

Cooking Spaghetti Squash Like a Pro

Most people cut spaghetti squash in half lengthwise before cooking, but if you cut it crosswise (or horizontally) you'll get longer "noodles." To cook spaghetti squash, cut off top and bottom and then cut into four pieces horizontally. Scoop out seeds and set each piece on a baking sheet. Bake at 400°F for 30 minutes. Pull spaghetti squash strands away from skin with a fork.

1. Turn broiler to high.

2. Heat olive oil in a large skillet over medium heat. Add garlic and cook until translucent, about 3 minutes. Add onions and mushrooms and cook until softened, about 4 minutes.

3. Add mayonnaise and cream cheese and stir until cheese is melted and mixture is smooth. Stir in salt, pepper, and nutmeg. Add Parmesan cheese and stir until smooth. Fold in baby spinach and artichoke hearts and continue stirring until cheese has melted.

4. Add cooked spaghetti squash to skillet and gently stir to coat. Transfer coated spaghetti squash to a 9" × 13" baking dish. Sprinkle mozzarella cheese on top.

5. Broil 3 minutes or until cheese is melted and bubbly.

6. Allow to cool and then divide into six equal portions. Transfer each portion to a separate airtight container and store in the refrigerator until ready to eat.

PER SERVING Calories: 291 | Fat: 25 g | Protein: 6 g | Sodium: 656 mg | Fiber: 4 g | Carbohydrates: 13 g | Sugar: 5 g

Vegan Walnut Hemp Fudge

This fudge lasts for 3 weeks in the refrigerator, so if you want to always have it on hand for a quick snack between meals, make a triple batch and incorporate it into your meal plan for 3 weeks.

INGREDIENTS | SERVES 6 (MAKES 12 PIECES)

⅓ cup no-sugar-added almond butter

3 tablespoons no-sugar-added coconut butter

⅓ cup raw cacao powder

¼ teaspoon liquid stevia

½ cup hemp seeds

½ cup crushed walnuts

What Is Coconut Butter?

Coconut butter, also called coconut manna, is a spread that's made from coconut meat. To make coconut butter, manufacturers blend or process the coconut meat until it reaches a creamy consistency, similar to that of peanut butter. It differs from coconut oil, which is the oil that has been removed from the coconut meat.

1. Combine almond butter and coconut butter in a small saucepan over low heat. Stir until melted and incorporated.

2. Stir in cacao powder, add liquid stevia, and keep stirring until smooth. Fold in hemp seeds and walnuts.

3. Pour mixture into an 8" × 8" baking dish lined with parchment paper and spread out evenly. Refrigerate until hardened, about 2 hours.

4. Cut into twelve equal-sized squares and transfer two squares to each of six snack bags or airtight containers. Store in the refrigerator until ready to eat.

PER SERVING Calories: 265 | Fat: 24 g | Protein: 8 g | Sodium: 61 mg | Fiber: 6 g | Carbohydrates: 10 g | Sugar: 2 g

Garlicky Kale and Mushrooms

This recipe calls for baby kale, which tends to be less tough than regular kale and doesn't require any extra preparation like chopping. However, if you can't find baby kale, you can use any type of kale; just chop it into small pieces before adding it to the pan. This will keep up to 1 week in the refrigerator.

INGREDIENTS | SERVES 6

2 tablespoons olive oil

4 cloves garlic, minced

1 large yellow onion, peeled and diced

½ cup sliced white mushrooms

6 cups baby kale

1 teaspoon salt

½ teaspoon freshly ground black pepper

⅛ teaspoon ground nutmeg

1. Heat olive oil over medium heat in a large skillet. Add garlic and cook until fragrant, about 3 minutes. Add onion and mushrooms and cook until softened, about 4 minutes.

2. Add kale and let it start to wilt. Add spices and stir to incorporate.

3. Remove from heat and allow to cool. Divide into six equal portions and store each portion in an airtight container in the refrigerator until ready to eat.

PER SERVING Calories: 64 | Fat: 5 g | Protein: 2 g | Sodium: 395 mg | Fiber: 1 g | Carbohydrates: 5 g | Sugar: 1 g

Spicy Broccoli Salad

This recipe uses raw broccoli, which will soften a bit from the vinegar and oil as it sits and marinates in the refrigerator. If you prefer to cook your broccoli, you can lightly steam it (no more than 5 minutes) and then follow the recipe as written. This salad will last up to 1 week in the refrigerator.

INGREDIENTS | SERVES 6

2 tablespoons avocado oil

3 tablespoons coconut aminos

3 tablespoons red curry paste

3 tablespoons lemon juice

¼ teaspoon salt

¼ teaspoon freshly ground black pepper

6 cups broccoli florets, chopped into bite-sized pieces

3 tablespoons sesame seeds

6 tablespoons chopped almonds

3 tablespoons chopped green onions

1. Combine avocado oil, coconut aminos, red curry paste, lemon juice, salt, and pepper in a large bowl and whisk to mix well.

2. Add remaining ingredients and toss to incorporate and coat completely.

3. Divide into six equal portions and transfer each portion to an airtight container. Store in the refrigerator until ready to eat.

PER SERVING Calories: 157 | Fat: 12 g | Protein: 6 g | Sodium: 495 mg | Fiber: 4 g | Carbohydrates: 11 g | Sugar: 3 g

CHAPTER 8

Salads

Mason Jar Cobb Salad

Mason jars are a great meal prepping tool because they're glass, they seal tightly to keep everything fresh, and the quart jars are the perfect size for a filling salad. Although you can use any Mason jar, wide-mouth jars are the easiest to fill quickly and without a mess. These salads will last up to 1 week in your refrigerator.

INGREDIENTS | SERVES 6

12 tablespoons Ranch Dressing (Chapter 9)

3 cups shredded canned chicken breast

3 cups chopped avocado

3 cups halved cherry tomatoes

6 large hard-boiled eggs, chopped

6 tablespoons blue cheese

6 tablespoons crumbled no-sugar-added bacon

6 cups chopped romaine lettuce

Layering the Perfect Mason Jar Salad

When layering Mason jar salad, you always want to put the dressing on the bottom, then layer it according to weight. The heaviest ingredients go in first, followed by the medium-weight ingredients, and then the lettuce or greens you're using. This keeps everything nicely separated so that your greens stay crispy until you're ready to eat them.

1. Scoop 2 tablespoons Ranch Dressing into the bottom of six Mason jars.

2. Layer ½ cup chicken breast, ½ cup avocado, ½ cup cherry tomatoes, 1 hard-boiled egg, 1 tablespoon blue cheese, and 1 tablespoon bacon in each Mason jar. Top each jar with 1 cup lettuce.

3. Cover jars and refrigerate for up to 1 week. When ready to eat, shake jar vigorously with lid on it until ingredients are combined.

PER SERVING   Calories: 678 | Fat: 51 g | Protein: 40 g | Sodium: 1,130 mg | Fiber: 7 g | Carbohydrates: 15 g | Sugar: 5 g

Bacon Broccoli Salad

Because this broccoli salad doesn't require you to cook the broccoli, you can throw it together in minutes. You can keep it in the refrigerator for 1 week, and the taste develops even more as it sits.

INGREDIENTS | SERVES 6

1 large head broccoli, cut into bite-sized florets

½ cup halved cherry tomatoes

8 ounces sharp Cheddar cheese, finely diced

½ cup chopped red onion

8 slices cooked no-sugar-added bacon, chopped

1 cup Basic Mayonnaise (Chapter 9)

¼ cup granulated erythritol

2 tablespoons white vinegar

1. Place broccoli in a large bowl.

2. Add tomatoes, cheese, onion, and bacon and toss to combine.

3. In a separate small bowl, combine mayonnaise, erythritol, and vinegar and stir to combine. Pour mayonnaise mixture over broccoli mixture and toss to coat evenly.

4. Divide into six equal portions and transfer each portion into a separate airtight container. Store in the refrigerator until ready to eat.

PER SERVING Calories: 157 | Fat: 12 g | Protein: 6 g | Sodium: 495 mg | Fiber: 4 g | Carbohydrates: 11 g | Sugar: 3 g

Avocado Tuna Salad

This tuna salad is great on its own or you can combine it with Cloud Bread (Chapter 15) or some cucumber slices. If you pair it with cucumber slices, wait to slice the cucumber until the day you're ready to eat it so it stays crispy. This salad will last in the refrigerator up to 1 week.

INGREDIENTS | SERVES 6

3 (5-ounce) cans tuna, packed in water

2 large avocados, pitted, peeled, and chopped

2 large hard-boiled eggs, chopped

3 tablespoons Basic Mayonnaise (Chapter 9)

3 tablespoons minced onion

2 tablespoons minced celery

½ teaspoon salt

¼ teaspoon freshly ground black pepper

⅛ teaspoon paprika

1. Combine all ingredients in a medium bowl and stir until combined.

2. Divide into six equal portions and store in the refrigerator in separate airtight containers until ready to eat.

PER SERVING Calories: 321 | Fat: 22 g | Protein: 23 g | Sodium: 554 mg | Fiber: 5 g | Carbohydrates: 6 g | Sugar: 1 g

Strawberry Fields Mason Jar Salad

This salad is vegan friendly as written. You can add a little bit of crumbled feta cheese for some salty flavor to turn it into a vegetarian-friendly salad. These salad jars will last up to 1 week in the refrigerator.

INGREDIENTS | SERVES 6

12 tablespoons Green Goddess Dressing (Chapter 9)

6 tablespoons chopped walnuts

6 tablespoons minced red onion

1½ cups chopped cucumber

6 tablespoons chopped avocado

6 large strawberries, chopped

6 cups chopped spinach

1. Scoop 2 tablespoons Green Goddess Dressing into the bottom of six Mason jars.

2. Layer 1 tablespoon walnuts, 1 tablespoon red onion, ¼ cup cucumber, 1 tablespoon avocado, and 1 strawberry in each Mason jar. Top each jar with 1 cup spinach.

3. Cover each jar and store in refrigerator for up to 1 week. When ready to eat, shake jar vigorously with lid on it until ingredients are combined.

PER SERVING Calories: 229 | Fat: 20 g | Protein: 3 g | Sodium: 293 mg | Fiber: 2 g | Carbohydrates: 11 g | Sugar: 7 g

Thai Chicken Mason Jar Salad

If you have frozen Easy Shredded Chicken (Chapter 13) on hand, you can use it in this recipe—and there's no need to thaw! Just assemble the salad with frozen chicken and allow it to thaw naturally in the refrigerator over the course of the week.

INGREDIENTS | SERVES 6

12 tablespoons Thai Peanut Sauce (Chapter 9)

3 cups shredded chicken

6 tablespoons minced red onion

6 tablespoons shredded carrots

6 tablespoons chopped peanuts

1½ cups chopped cucumber

6 cups chopped iceberg lettuce

1. Scoop 2 tablespoons Thai Peanut Sauce into the bottom of six Mason jars.

2. Layer ½ cup chicken, 1 tablespoon red onion, 1 tablespoon carrots, 1 tablespoon peanuts, and ¼ cup cucumber in each Mason jar. Top each jar with 1 cup iceberg lettuce.

3. Cover each jar and store in refrigerator for up to 1 week. When ready to eat, shake jar vigorously with lid on it until ingredients are combined.

PER SERVING Calories: 493 | Fat: 36 g | Protein: 35 g | Sodium: 130 mg | Fiber: 2 g | Carbohydrates: 6 g | Sugar: 3 g

Oodles of Zoodles Mason Jar Salad

There is no need to cook your zucchini noodles. The dressing will soften them just enough to make them tender but still give you a nice crunch. This salad will keep up to 1 week in the refrigerator.

INGREDIENTS | SERVES 6

12 tablespoons Cilantro Lime Dressing (Chapter 9)

1½ cups canned shredded chicken

6 tablespoons sesame seeds

6 tablespoons chopped cashews

1½ cups chopped red bell pepper

6 cups spiralized zucchini

1. Scoop 2 tablespoons Cilantro Lime Dressing into the bottom of six Mason jars.

2. Layer ¼ cup chicken, 1 tablespoon sesame seeds, 1 tablespoon cashews, ¼ cup bell pepper, and 1 cup zucchini in each Mason jar.

3. Cover each jar and store in refrigerator for up to 1 week. When ready to eat, shake jar vigorously with lid on it until ingredients are combined.

PER SERVING   Calories: 416 | Fat: 32 g | Protein: 19 g | Sodium: 253 mg | Fiber: 4 g | Carbohydrates: 16 g | Sugar: 6 g

Chicken Cauliflower Mason Jar Salad

If you prefer your cauliflower cooked, use the pressure cooker riced cauliflower method and add the cooked cauliflower to your Mason jar salad after it cools. This salad will keep up to 1 week in the refrigerator.

INGREDIENTS | SERVES 6

12 tablespoons Bacon Chipotle Ranch Dressing (Chapter 9)

1½ cups chopped cooked chicken

6 tablespoons chopped scallions

1½ cups chopped yellow bell pepper

6 tablespoons minced cilantro

1½ cups raw riced cauliflower

1. Scoop 2 tablespoons Bacon Chipotle Ranch Dressing into the bottom of six Mason jars.

2. Layer each jar with ¼ cup chicken, 1 tablespoon scallions, ¼ cup bell pepper, 1 tablespoon cilantro, and ¼ cup cauliflower rice.

3. Cover each jar and store in refrigerator for up to 1 week. When ready to eat, shake jar vigorously with lid on it until ingredients are combined.

PER SERVING   Calories: 201 | Fat: 16 g | Protein: 11 g | Sodium: 140 mg | Fiber: 1 g | Carbohydrates: 4 g | Sugar: 2 g

Greek Mason Jar Salad

This salad gives you all the flavors of a gyro without the extra carbohydrates. If you want it even more authentic, use cooked ground lamb in place of the chicken. You can keep this salad up to 1 week in the refrigerator.

INGREDIENTS | SERVES 6

12 tablespoons Tzatziki Sauce (Chapter 9)

1½ cups cooked cubed chicken

6 tablespoons chopped Kalamata olives

1½ cups chopped cucumber

6 tablespoons crumbled feta cheese

6 cups romaine lettuce

Homemade Greek Dressing

If you prefer an oily dressing to a creamy one, you can replace the Tzatziki Sauce in this recipe with a quick Greek dressing. To make, combine ½ cup olive oil, 2 minced garlic cloves, 2 teaspoons Dijon mustard, 2 tablespoons lemon juice, 4 tablespoons red wine vinegar, ¼ teaspoon dried basil, ¼ teaspoon dried oregano, and ¼ teaspoon salt in a small bowl and whisk to mix well.

1. Scoop 2 tablespoons Tzatziki Sauce into the bottom of six Mason jars.

2. Layer ¼ cup chicken, 1 tablespoon olives, ¼ cup cucumber, and 1 tablespoon feta cheese in each jar. Top each jar with 1 cup romaine lettuce.

3. Cover each jar and store in refrigerator for up to 1 week. When ready to eat, shake jar vigorously with lid on it until ingredients are combined.

PER SERVING   Calories: 129 | Fat: 6 g | Protein: 13 g | Sodium: 165 mg | Fiber: 1 g | Carbohydrates: 6 g | Sugar: 3 g

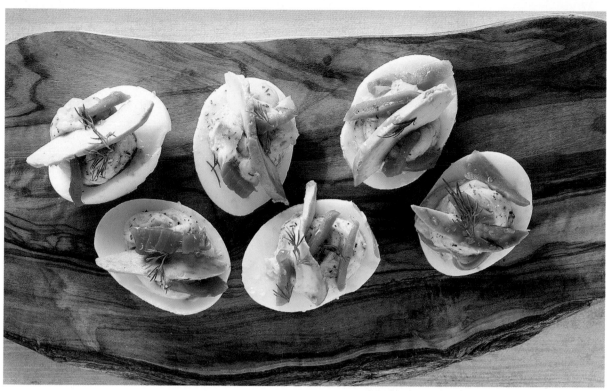

Smoked Salmon Deviled Eggs (Chapter 3)

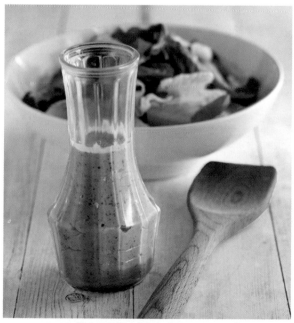

Green Goddess Dressing (Chapter 9)

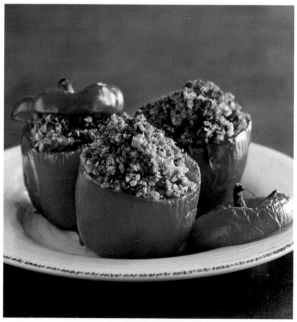

Sausage-Stuffed Peppers (Chapter 12)

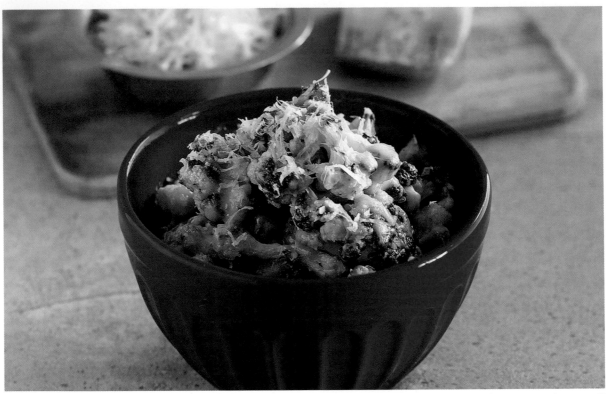

Cauliflower Mac 'n' Cheese (Chapter 7)

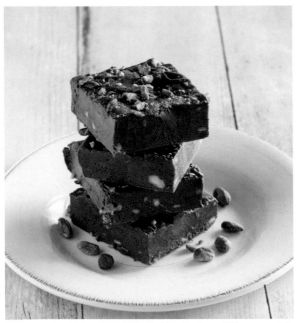

Pistachio Fudge (Chapter 16)

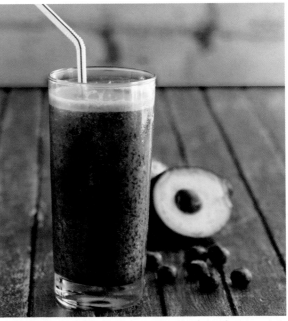

Blueberry Vanilla Smoothie Packs (Chapter 14)

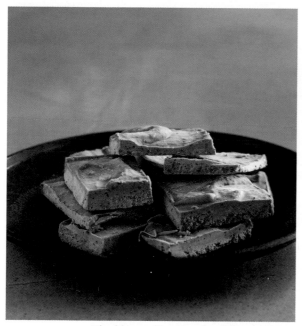

Blackberry Fat Bombs (Chapter 15)

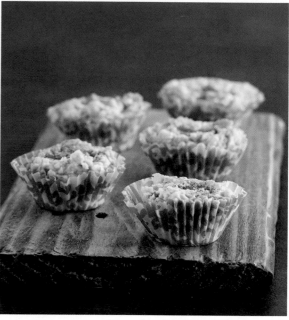

Pumpkin Pie Bites (Chapter 16)

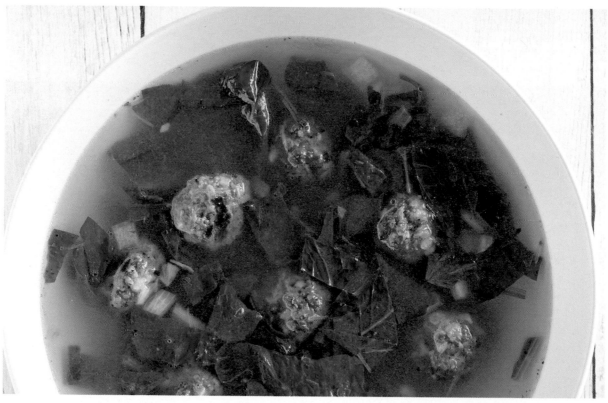

Italian Wedding Soup (Chapter 13)

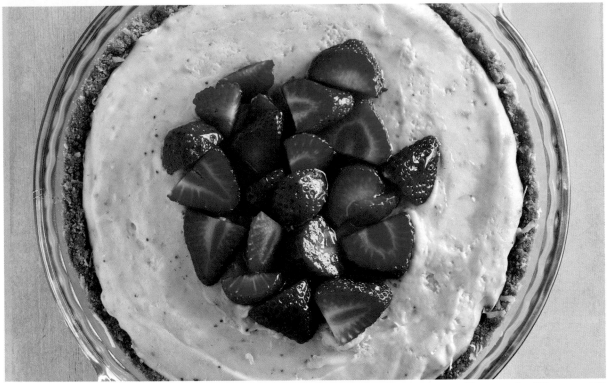

Strawberry Cheesecake (Chapter 16)

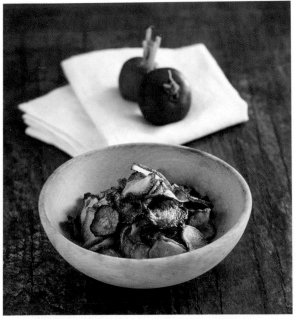

Salt and Vinegar Radish Chips (Chapter 10)

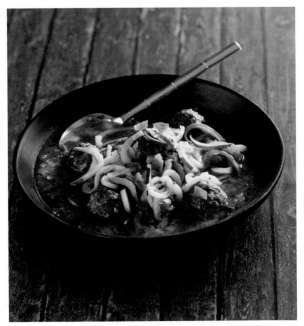

Meatball Zoodle Soup (Chapter 5)

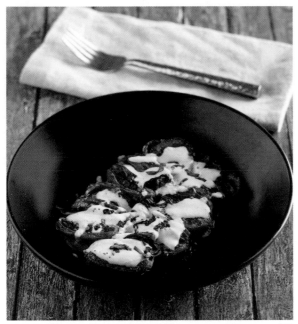

Mozzarella and Basil Tomatoes (Chapter 10)

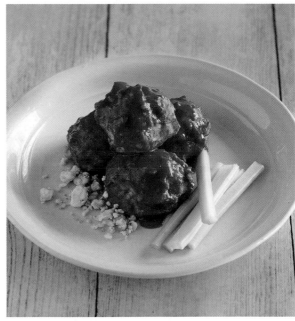

Buffalo Chicken Meatballs (Chapter 4)

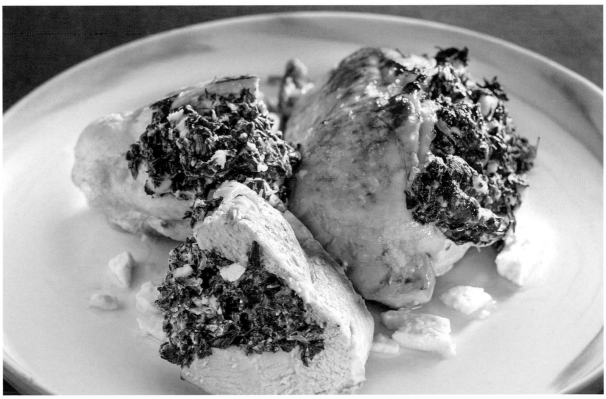

Spinach-and-Feta-Stuffed Chicken Breast
(Chapter 4)

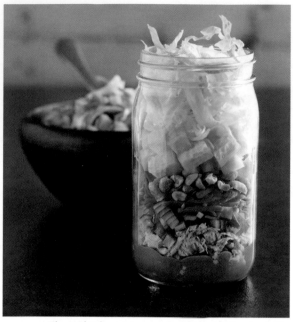

Thai Chicken Mason Jar Salad (Chapter 8)

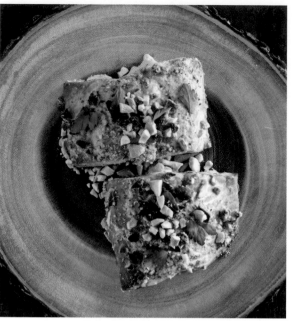

Dijon-Rubbed Salmon (Chapter 17)

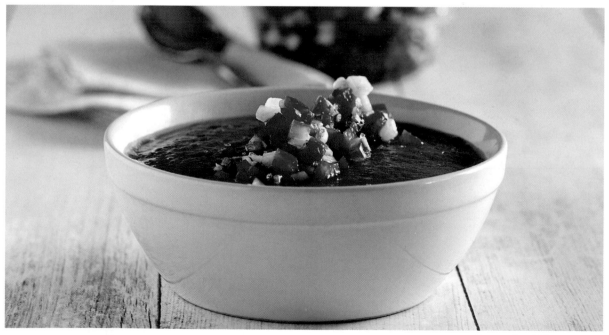

Gazpacho (Chapter 11)

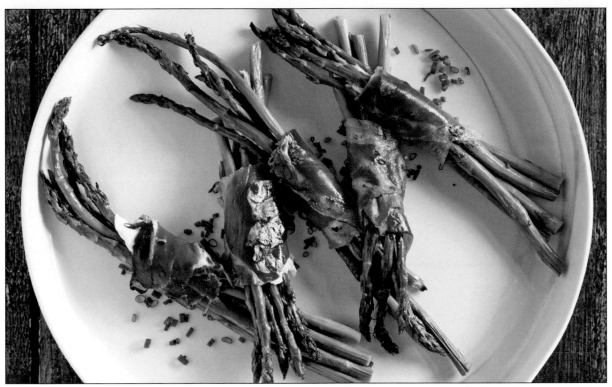

Prosciutto-Wrapped Asparagus (Chapter 17)

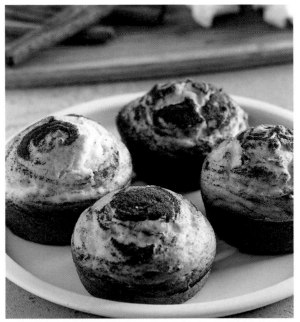

Cinnamon Swirl Muffins (Chapter 3)

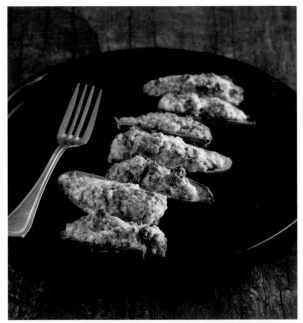

Sausage Jalapeño Poppers (Chapter 6)

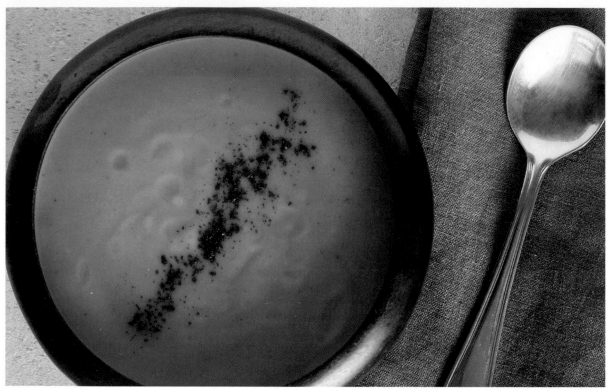

Spicy Pumpkin Soup (Chapter 11)

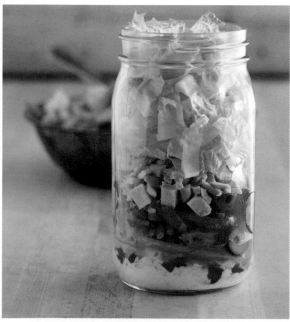

Colorful Veggie Mason Jar Salad (Chapter 8)

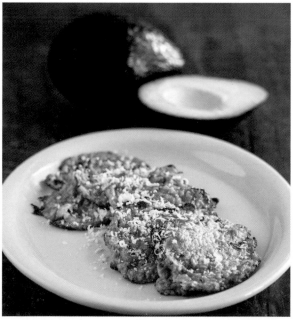

Avocado Chips (Chapter 15)

Broccoli Tuna Mason Jar Salad

You can use raw or steamed broccoli for this salad, based on your own preferences. Raw broccoli holds up better in the refrigerator and will soften when mixed with the dressing. This salad will keep in the refrigerator up to 1 week.

INGREDIENTS | SERVES 6

12 tablespoons Creamy Mustard Dressing (Chapter 9)

3 (5-ounce) cans tuna, packed in water

3 cups chopped broccoli

6 tablespoons minced red onion

1½ cups tomatoes, chopped and seeded

6 large hard-boiled eggs, chopped

1. Scoop 2 tablespoons Creamy Mustard Dressing into the bottom of six Mason jars.

2. Layer ½ can tuna, ½ cup broccoli, 1 tablespoon onion, ¼ cup tomatoes, and 1 hard-boiled egg in each jar.

3. Cover each jar and store in refrigerator for up to 1 week. When ready to eat, shake jar vigorously with lid on it until ingredients are combined.

PER SERVING   Calories: 357 | Fat: 24 g | Protein: 28 g | Sodium: 380 mg | Fiber: 2 g | Carbohydrates: 6 g | Sugar: 3 g

Taco Mason Jar Salad

Allow the taco meat to cool fully before assembling your Mason jars. If you put it in while it's hot, the steam will cause the other ingredients to cook and wilt, and the shelf life won't be as long. If you prepare it properly, it will keep in the refrigerator up to 1 week.

INGREDIENTS | SERVES 6

6 tablespoons Enchilada Sauce (Chapter 9)

3 cups taco meat

6 tablespoons minced green onion

1½ cups tomatoes, chopped and seeded

12 tablespoons chopped avocado

6 tablespoons shredded Cheddar cheese

1½ cups raw cauliflower rice

1. Scoop 1 tablespoon Enchilada Sauce into the bottom of six Mason jars.

2. Layer ½ cup taco meat, 1 tablespoon green onion, ¼ cup tomato, 2 tablespoons avocado, 1 tablespoon Cheddar cheese, and ¼ cup cauliflower rice in each Mason jar.

3. Cover each jar and store in refrigerator for up to 1 week. When ready to eat, shake jar vigorously with lid on it until ingredients are combined.

PER SERVING   Calories: 342 | Fat: 20 g | Protein: 33 g | Sodium: 164 mg | Fiber: 2.5 g | Carbohydrates: 5 g | Sugar: 2 g

Chipotle Chicken and Kale Mason Jar Salad

Baby kale tends to be less tough than regular kale, but if you can't find any or have regular kale on hand, you can use that instead. When ready to eat, shake the jar and allow the kale to sit in the dressing for a little while to soften before eating. This salad will keep in the refrigerator up to 1 week.

INGREDIENTS | SERVES 6

12 tablespoons Bacon Chipotle Ranch Dressing (Chapter 9)

1½ cups cubed, cooked chicken

6 tablespoons chopped cooked no-sugar-added bacon

6 tablespoons chopped walnuts

6 tablespoons sunflower seeds

1½ cups chopped avocado

6 cups baby kale

Nutrient-Rich Sunflower Seeds

Sunflower seeds have high levels of phytosterols, compounds that help lower blood cholesterol and help boost heart health. A quarter cup of sunflower seeds also provides 60 percent of your daily needs for vitamin E and 25 percent of your daily magnesium—a nutrient many adults are deficient in.

1. Scoop 2 tablespoons Bacon Chipotle Ranch Dressing into the bottom of six Mason jars.

2. Layer ½ cup chicken, 1 tablespoon bacon, 1 tablespoon walnuts, 1 tablespoon sunflower seeds, and ¼ cup avocado in each jar. Top each jar with 1 cup kale.

3. Cover each jar and store in refrigerator for up to 1 week. When ready to eat, shake jar vigorously with lid on it until ingredients are combined.

PER SERVING   Calories: 466 | Fat: 41 g | Protein: 18 g | Sodium: 171 mg | Fiber: 4 g | Carbohydrates: 8 g | Sugar: 1 g

Greek Zoodle Mason Jar Salad

This salad is best assembled in a one-quart Mason jar. This provides enough room for the zucchini noodles without crushing them and gives you room to shake everything when you're ready to eat it. It will last up to 1 week in the refrigerator.

INGREDIENTS | SERVES 6

12 tablespoons Green Goddess Dressing (Chapter 9)

1½ cups chopped celery

1½ cups chopped cherry tomatoes

6 tablespoons chopped Kalamata olives

1½ cups roasted red peppers

3 cups spiralized zucchini

6 tablespoons feta cheese

3 cups baby spinach

1. Scoop 2 tablespoons Green Goddess Dressing into the bottom of six Mason jars.

2. Layer ¼ cup celery, ¼ cup tomato, 1 tablespoon olives, ¼ cup red peppers, ½ cup zucchini, and 1 tablespoon feta cheese in each jar. Top each jar with ½ cup spinach.

3. Cover each jar and store in refrigerator for up to 1 week. When ready to eat, shake jar vigorously with lid on it until ingredients are combined.

PER SERVING   Calories: 192 | Fat: 16 g | Protein: 4 g | Sodium: 133 mg | Fiber: 3 g | Carbohydrates: 10 g | Sugar: 5 g

Colorful Veggie Mason Jar Salad

You can change this salad up by adding any low-carb vegetables that are left over in your refrigerator after meal prepping. These vegetable medley Mason jar salads are a great way to clear out your refrigerator and reduce waste. You can keep this salad in the refrigerator up to 1 week.

INGREDIENTS | SERVES 6

12 tablespoons Ranch Dressing (Chapter 9)

¾ cup chopped yellow bell pepper

¾ cup chopped orange bell pepper

¾ cup roasted red pepper

6 tablespoons chopped black olives

¾ cup chopped avocado

¾ cup chopped cashews

6 cups romaine lettuce

1. Scoop 2 tablespoons Ranch Dressing into the bottom of six Mason jars.

2. Layer ⅛ cup yellow peppers, ⅛ cup orange peppers, ⅛ cup red peppers, 1 tablespoon black olives, ⅛ cup avocado, and ⅛ cup cashews in each jar. Top each jar with 1 cup romaine lettuce.

3. Cover each jar and store in refrigerator for up to 1 week. When ready to eat, shake jar vigorously with lid on it until ingredients are combined.

PER SERVING   Calories: 336 | Fat: 26 g | Protein: 10 g | Sodium: 117 mg | Fiber: 5 g | Carbohydrates: 12 g | Sugar: 4 g

Cilantro Lime Zoodle Mason Jar Salad

Frozen baby shrimp is great to have in your freezer when you're meal prepping because it's the most inexpensive shrimp size, and it's an easy protein source that thaws quickly. Watch for sales and stock up when you find one. You can keep this salad up to 3 days in the refrigerator.

INGREDIENTS | SERVES 6

12 tablespoons Cilantro Lime Dressing (Chapter 9)

6 cups spiralized zucchini

3 cups cooked baby shrimp

6 tablespoons chopped scallions

6 tablespoons chopped cilantro

¾ cup crumbled feta

The Lowdown on Scallions

Scallions go by several different names, including green onions, spring onions, and Welsh onions. They belong to the *Allium* plant genus, which also includes garlic, onions, leeks, shallots, and chives. Both the green and white parts of the scallion can be used in cooking, but the green portion has a milder flavor and is typically consumed raw, while the white portion is stronger and generally cooked before eating.

1. Scoop 2 tablespoons Cilantro Lime Dressing into the bottom of six Mason jars.

2. Layer 1 cup zucchini, ½ cup shrimp, 1 tablespoon scallions, 1 tablespoon cilantro, and ⅛ cup feta in each jar.

3. Cover each jar and store in refrigerator up to 3 days. When ready to eat, shake jar vigorously with lid on it until ingredients are combined.

PER SERVING Calories: 251 | Fat: 18 g | Protein: 15 g | Sodium: 618 mg | Fiber: 2 g | Carbohydrates: 6 g | Sugar: 4 g

Blueberry Garden Mason Jar Salad

You can use frozen blueberries rather than fresh blueberries in this recipe. Throw the blueberries into the Mason jar frozen and let them thaw in the refrigerator as the week goes on. As the blueberries thaw, they'll create a juice that adds an extra sweet flavor to this salad. You can keep this salad in the refrigerator up to 1 week.

INGREDIENTS | SERVES 6

12 tablespoons Simple Salad Dressing (Chapter 9)

1½ cups shredded canned chicken

1½ cups blueberries

¾ cup sliced almonds

¾ cup raw sunflower seeds

¾ cup crumbled Gorgonzola cheese

6 cups baby spinach

1. Scoop 2 tablespoons Simple Salad Dressing into the bottom of six Mason jars.

2. Layer ¼ cup chicken, ¼ cup blueberries, ⅛ cup almonds, ⅛ cup sunflower seeds, and ⅛ cup Gorgonzola cheese in each jar. Top each jar with 1 cup baby spinach.

3. Cover each jar and store in refrigerator for up to 1 week. When ready to eat, shake jar vigorously with lid on it until ingredients are combined.

PER SERVING Calories: 458 | Fat: 36 g | Protein: 22 g | Sodium: 261 mg | Fiber: 5 g | Carbohydrates: 14 g | Sugar: 5 g

Caprese Mason Jar Salad

If it's easier for you, you can use shredded mozzarella cheese in this salad, but fresh mozzarella balls give a nice creamy texture that's worth the extra prep time. This salad will last 1 week in the refrigerator.

INGREDIENTS | SERVES 6

12 tablespoons balsamic vinegar

12 tablespoons olive oil

1½ cups halved cherry tomatoes

1½ cups fresh mozzarella balls, roughly chopped

1½ cups fresh basil

1½ cups chopped avocado

1. Put 2 tablespoons balsamic vinegar and 2 tablespoons olive oil in the bottom of each of six Mason jars.

2. Layer ¼ cup tomatoes, ¼ cup mozzarella, ¼ cup basil, and ¼ cup avocado in each jar.

3. Cover each jar and store in refrigerator for up to 1 week. When ready to eat, shake jar vigorously with lid on it until ingredients are combined.

PER SERVING Calories: 421 | Fat: 38 g | Protein: 8 g | Sodium: 188 mg | Fiber: 3 g | Carbohydrates: 11 g | Sugar: 6 g

Zesty Arugula Mason Jar Salad

When it comes to this salad, zesty is an understatement. If you want less of a kick, omit the jalapeños or swap the arugula for a less bitter green like spinach. This salad will keep in the refrigerator for 1 week.

INGREDIENTS | SERVES 6

6 tablespoons olive oil

6 tablespoons apple cider vinegar

6 tablespoons seeded and minced jalapeño

3 teaspoons minced garlic

3 cups cooked cubed chicken

¾ cup chopped green olives

¾ cup feta cheese

6 cups arugula

1. Put 1 tablespoon olive oil, 1 tablespoon vinegar, 1 tablespoon jalapeño, and ½ teaspoon garlic in the bottom of each of six Mason jars. Swirl the jar to combine.

2. Layer ½ cup chicken, ⅛ cup olives, and ⅛ cup feta in each jar. Top with 1 cup arugula.

3. Cover each jar and store in refrigerator for up to 1 week. When ready to eat, shake jar vigorously with lid on it until ingredients are combined.

PER SERVING Calories: 332 | Fat: 24 g | Protein: 23 g | Sodium: 362 mg | Fiber: 1 g | Carbohydrates: 4 g | Sugar: 1.5 g

Creamy Cucumber Salad

You can make this recipe dairy-free by swapping the sour cream and yogurt combo for ½ cup Basic Mayonnaise (Chapter 9). It will still last in the refrigerator for 1 week.

INGREDIENTS | SERVES 6

¼ cup sour cream

¼ cup full-fat plain Greek yogurt

2 tablespoons chopped fresh dill

1½ tablespoons olive oil

1 tablespoon lime juice

½ teaspoon garlic powder

½ teaspoon salt

¼ teaspoon freshly ground black pepper

6 cups chopped cucumber

1 small red onion, peeled and minced

1. Combine sour cream, yogurt, dill, olive oil, lime juice, garlic powder, salt, and pepper in a medium bowl. Mix until incorporated.

2. Add cucumber and onion and toss until evenly coated.

3. Divide into six equal portions and store each portion in a separate airtight container in the refrigerator until ready to eat.

PER SERVING Calories: 440 | Fat: 32 g | Protein: 13 g | Sodium: 923 mg | Fiber: 4.5 g | Carbohydrates: 20 g | Sugar: 8 g

Cauliflower and Herb Salad

This salad gives traditional potato salad a run for its money with only a fraction of the carbohydrates. This dish will keep up to 1 week in the refrigerator.

INGREDIENTS | SERVES 6

1 cup water

6 cups cauliflower florets

⅔ cup Basic Mayonnaise (Chapter 9)

¼ cup minced red onion

1 tablespoon white vinegar

1 teaspoon dry mustard powder

2 tablespoons lemon juice

1 teaspoon salt

½ teaspoon freshly ground black pepper

¼ cup chopped fresh dill

3 tablespoons chopped scallions

4 large hard-boiled eggs, chopped

1. Put water and cauliflower florets in a large pot and bring water to a boil. Reduce heat to medium, cover, and let cauliflower steam until softened but still slightly crisp, about 5 minutes. Transfer to a large bowl and allow to cool.

2. In a separate small bowl, combine mayonnaise, onion, vinegar, dry mustard, lemon juice, salt, pepper, and dill.

3. Pour mayonnaise mixture over cauliflower and toss to coat evenly. Sprinkle chopped scallions and eggs on top.

4. Divide into six equal portions and store each portion in a separate container in the refrigerator until ready to eat.

PER SERVING Calories: 256 | Fat: 23 g | Protein: 7 g | Sodium: 617 mg | Fiber: 3 g | Carbohydrates: 7 g | Sugar: 3 g

Cheeseburger Mason Jar Salad

If you don't typically put ketchup and mayonnaise on your cheeseburgers, you can replace those two ingredients with 12 tablespoons of the Bacon Chipotle Ranch Dressing (Chapter 9). The smoky flavor makes a nice addition to this Mason jar salad. You can keep this salad in the refrigerator up to 1 week.

INGREDIENTS | SERVES 6

6 tablespoons ketchup

6 tablespoons Basic Mayonnaise (Chapter 9)

3 cups cooked lean 85/15 ground beef

1½ cups tomatoes, chopped and seeded

¾ cup chopped pickles

¾ cup shredded Cheddar cheese

6 cups iceberg lettuce

1. Scoop 1 tablespoon ketchup and 1 tablespoon Basic Mayonnaise into the bottom of each of six Mason jars.

2. Layer ½ cup ground beef, ¼ cup tomatoes, ⅛ cup pickles, and ⅛ cup cheese in each jar. Top each jar with 1 cup lettuce.

3. Cover each jar and store in refrigerator for up to 1 week. When ready to eat, shake jar vigorously with lid on it until ingredients are combined.

PER SERVING Calories: 342 | Fat: 23 g | Protein: 19 g | Sodium: 485 mg | Fiber: 1.5 g | Carbohydrates: 13 g | Sugar: 9 g

Not Just Water

Iceberg lettuce is known for being mostly water, and that's true. The vegetable ties with cucumbers for the most water content of any vegetable at 96 percent; however, iceberg lettuce offers more than that. In addition to contributing to your hydration needs, 1 cup of iceberg lettuce provides 2 grams of fiber and 7 percent of your daily needs for vitamin A.

CHAPTER 9

Sauces and Dressings

Basic Mayonnaise

Since this recipe calls for raw egg yolks, it's best to use really fresh eggs so you can store it for a week and use it when needed. Your local farm is best, but if you don't have access to a farm, use organic eggs from the grocery store and find the ones with the latest sell-by date. This will last 1 week in the refrigerator.

INGREDIENTS | SERVES 6

2 large egg yolks

Juice from ½ medium lemon (about 3 teaspoons)

1 cup avocado oil (or light olive oil)

1 teaspoon dry mustard powder

¼ teaspoon salt

1. Combine egg yolks with lemon juice in a medium bowl and allow to come to room temperature. Once mixture reaches room temperature, add oil, mustard powder, and salt.

2. Use an immersion blender to combine mixture. Store in the refrigerator until ready to use.

PER SERVING Calories: 340 | Fat: 37 g | Protein: 1 g | Sodium: 108 mg | Fiber: 0 g | Carbohydrates: 0 g | Sugar: 0 g

Ranch Dressing

Make this ranch dressing at the same time you make your Basic Mayonnaise (see recipe in this chapter) so you can keep track of the use-by date. It's helpful to store in a glass jar with a piece of tape that marks the date by which you should use it. It will last for up to 1 week in the refrigerator.

INGREDIENTS | SERVES 6

½ teaspoon dried parsley

½ teaspoon dried dill

½ teaspoon dried chives

¼ teaspoon garlic powder

¼ teaspoon onion powder

¼ teaspoon salt

¼ teaspoon freshly ground black pepper

½ cup Basic Mayonnaise (see recipe in this chapter)

½ cup sour cream

1. Mix all herbs and spices together in a small bowl. In a separate medium bowl, combine mayonnaise and sour cream and stir until incorporated.

2. Add herb mixture to mayonnaise mixture and stir to combine. Store in a glass jar with a lid in the refrigerator.

PER SERVING Calories: 164 | Fat: 17 g | Protein: 0 g | Sodium: 209 mg | Fiber: 0 g | Carbohydrates: 1 g | Sugar: 0 g

Coconut Sour Cream

This recipe requires some planning ahead, since the coconut milk must be chilled. Keep that in mind when using it for your recipes. Store in the refrigerator up to 1 week.

INGREDIENTS | SERVES 12

1 (13.5-ounce) can full-fat coconut milk

1 tablespoon fresh lemon juice

½ tablespoon apple cider vinegar

1. Place coconut milk in refrigerator and allow to chill overnight. In the morning, open can, carefully scoop out "cream" that's hardened on top, and place in a blender or food processor. Set liquid aside.

2. Add lemon juice and vinegar to coconut cream and blend until smooth.

3. Store in an airtight container in the refrigerator until ready to use.

PER SERVING Calories: 74 | Fat: 8 g | Protein: 0.5 g | Sodium: 5 mg | Fiber: 0 g | Carbohydrates: 1 g | Sugar: 0 g

Bacon Chipotle Ranch Dressing

Like the Ranch Dressing in this chapter, it's best to make this dressing along with a fresh batch of Basic Mayonnaise so you can keep track of your use-by dates. Consider this when mapping out your meal plan for the week. This dressing will keep in the refrigerator up to 1 week.

INGREDIENTS | SERVES 6

⅓ cup Basic Mayonnaise (see recipe in this chapter)

⅓ cup full-fat coconut milk

3 pieces no-sugar-added bacon, cooked and chopped

2 tablespoons minced chipotle peppers in adobo sauce

2 cloves garlic, minced

1 teaspoon dried dill

½ teaspoon dried parsley

½ teaspoon dried chives

¼ teaspoon salt

¼ teaspoon freshly ground black pepper

1. Place all ingredients in a blender or food processor. Blend until smooth.

2. Store in an airtight container in the refrigerator.

PER SERVING Calories: 173 | Fat: 17 g | Protein: 2.5 g | Sodium: 261 mg | Fiber: 0 g | Carbohydrates: 1.5 g | Sugar: 0 g

Creamy Blue Cheese Dressing

The high moisture content of blue cheese adds a decadent creaminess and rich flavor to this dressing. You can store it in one container in the refrigerator for up to 1 week and use it as needed or divide it into smaller portions if you want to take it with you on the go.

INGREDIENTS | SERVES 6

¾ cup blue cheese crumbles

2 tablespoons Basic Mayonnaise (see recipe in this chapter)

⅓ cup sour cream

2 tablespoons full-fat coconut milk

1 clove garlic, minced

1 tablespoon lemon juice

¼ teaspoon salt

⅛ teaspoon freshly ground black pepper

1. Place blue cheese in a small bowl and use a fork to mash. Add mayonnaise and continue mashing to form a paste. Add sour cream and coconut milk and stir to combine.

2. Add remaining ingredients and stir until incorporated.

3. Store in an airtight container in the refrigerator.

PER SERVING Calories: 123 | Fat: 12 g | Protein: 4 g | Sodium: 322 mg | Fiber: 0 g | Carbohydrates: 1 g | Sugar: 0 g

Thai Peanut Sauce

If you can't eat peanuts, you can use smooth almond butter in this recipe for a similar effect. If you can't tolerate any nuts, try sunflower seed butter instead. This sauce will last in the refrigerator up to 1 week.

INGREDIENTS | SERVES 6

½ cup no-sugar-added creamy peanut butter

⅔ cup full-fat coconut milk

1 teaspoon minced ginger

1 teaspoon minced garlic

1 tablespoon chopped jalapeño

1 tablespoon granulated erythritol

1 teaspoon coconut aminos

1 teaspoon sesame oil

1. Combine all ingredients in a blender or food processor and blend until smooth.

2. Store in an airtight container in the refrigerator.

PER SERVING Calories: 186 | Fat: 17 g | Protein: 5 g | Sodium: 118 mg | Fiber: 1 g | Carbohydrates: 8 g | Sugar: 2 g

Creamy Mustard Dressing

If you want to extend the shelf life of this dressing and you're able to tolerate dairy, you can replace the mayonnaise with sour cream or plain yogurt. This dressing will keep in the refrigerator up to 1 week.

INGREDIENTS | SERVES 6

¼ cup Basic Mayonnaise (see recipe in this chapter)
2 teaspoons dry mustard powder
¼ cup extra-virgin olive oil
2 cloves garlic, minced
2 tablespoons fresh lemon juice
1 tablespoon fresh chopped parsley
1 teaspoon dried oregano
½ teaspoon onion powder

1. Combine all ingredients together in a glass jar with a lid. Shake to combine.

2. Store covered in the refrigerator.

PER SERVING   Calories: 149 | Fat: 16 g | Protein: 0 g | Sodium: 72 mg | Fiber: 0 g | Carbohydrates: 1 g | Sugar: 0 g

Simple Salad Dressing

This dressing can be kept at room temperature for up to 3 weeks; however, if you're not going to use it often, it's best to store it in the refrigerator. You can make it your own by adding any combination of fresh herbs or spices.

INGREDIENTS | SERVES 6

¾ cup extra-virgin olive oil
2 tablespoons apple cider vinegar
¼ teaspoon salt
¼ teaspoon freshly ground black pepper
1 tablespoon chopped fresh parsley
1 teaspoon minced garlic

Combine all ingredients in a glass jar with a lid. Shake to combine.

PER SERVING   Calories: 240 | Fat: 27 g | Protein: 0 g | Sodium: 98 mg | Fiber: 0 g | Carbohydrates: 0 g | Sugar: 0 g

Storing Oil Properly

It's best to store oils in a cool, dark place. Don't store oil on the counter or near the stove. Both light and heat break down the fats and cause them to go rancid more quickly. This not only affects the taste, but also diminishes the nutritional quality.

Green Goddess Dressing

The avocado gives this dressing a creamy texture rather than an oily one, but it does shorten the shelf life. If you want this dressing to last longer, you can omit the avocado and increase the avocado oil slightly. Otherwise, plan your meals so that you use it up in 1 week.

INGREDIENTS | SERVES 6

½ cup fresh basil

1 medium avocado, pitted and peeled

¼ cup avocado oil

¼ cup water

2 tablespoons apple cider vinegar

2 cloves garlic, minced

2 tablespoons fresh chives

½ teaspoon salt

¼ teaspoon freshly ground black pepper

1. Combine all ingredients in a blender or food processor and blend until smooth.

2. Store in an airtight container in the refrigerator.

PER SERVING Calories: 137 | Fat: 14 g | Protein: 1 g | Sodium: 197 mg | Fiber: 2 g | Carbohydrates: 3 g | Sugar: 0 g

Tzatziki Sauce

Straining the excess water from the cucumber is extremely important to ensure that you don't wind up with a watery tzatziki sauce. Don't skip this step. This sauce will last in the refrigerator up to 2 weeks.

INGREDIENTS | SERVES 12

½ large English cucumber, peeled and grated

2 cups full-fat plain Greek yogurt

⅓ cup chopped fresh dill

2 cloves garlic, minced

1 tablespoon extra-virgin olive oil

Juice from ½ medium lemon (about 1 tablespoon)

½ teaspoon salt

1. Place grated cucumber in a cheesecloth or nut bag. Squeeze out as much excess moisture as you can.

2. Combine strained cucumber with the rest of the ingredients and allow to sit overnight in the refrigerator in a sealed container before serving.

3. Store in an airtight container in the refrigerator.

PER SERVING Calories: 35 | Fat: 4 g | Protein: 5 g | Sodium: 30 mg | Fiber: 0 g | Carbohydrates: 3 g | Sugar: 2 g

Cilantro Lime Dressing

You can store this dressing at room temperature up to 3 weeks. The dressing will become spicier as it sits as the lime juice pulls out the capsaicin from the jalapeño pepper.

INGREDIENTS | SERVES 6

¾ cup avocado oil

3 cloves garlic, minced

½ cup fresh cilantro

Juice from 1 large lime (about 2 tablespoons)

¼ teaspoon salt

1 small jalapeño, seeded

1. Add all ingredients to a blender and blend until smooth.

2. Transfer to an airtight container.

PER SERVING Calories: 243 | Fat: 27 g | Protein: 0 g | Sodium: 97 mg | Fiber: 0 g | Carbohydrates: 0 g | Sugar: 0 g

Beyond the Spice

Research shows that capsaicin, the spicy compound in chili peppers, can contribute to weight loss by boosting metabolism, diminishing appetite, and helping burn fat.

Spicy Dill Sauce

As is, you can store this spicy sauce in the refrigerator for 1 week. If you want to store it 2 weeks, use 1 cup of Greek yogurt and no mayonnaise in the recipe.

INGREDIENTS | SERVES 6

½ cup full-fat Greek yogurt

½ cup Basic Mayonnaise (see recipe in this chapter)

Juice from 1 medium lime

1 medium jalapeño, seeded and minced

½ teaspoon dried oregano

½ teaspoon dried dill

½ teaspoon ground cumin

½ teaspoon cayenne pepper

1. Combine yogurt and mayonnaise in a small bowl and stir until combined. Add lime juice and stir until incorporated. Add spices and herbs and mix well.

2. Store in an airtight container in the refrigerator.

PER SERVING Calories: 145 | Fat: 18 g | Protein: 3 g | Sodium: 118 mg | Fiber: 0 g | Carbohydrates: 3 g | Sugar: 1 g

Caesar Salad Dressing

The anchovy paste in this dressing makes it an authentic Caesar, but if you'd rather leave it out, just add a little more salt. You can keep this dressing in the refrigerator up to 1 week.

INGREDIENTS | SERVES 6

¾ cup Basic Mayonnaise (see recipe in this chapter)

1 clove garlic

1 tablespoon fresh lemon juice

½ teaspoon dry mustard powder

1 teaspoon anchovy paste

1 teaspoon white vinegar

¼ teaspoon salt

2 tablespoons grated Parmesan cheese

1. Add all ingredients except Parmesan cheese to a blender or food processor and blend until smooth.

2. Stir in Parmesan cheese.

3. Store in an airtight container in the refrigerator.

PER SERVING Calories: 208 | Fat: 22 g | Protein: 1 g | Sodium: 296 mg | Fiber: 0 g | Carbohydrates: 2 g | Sugar: 0 g

Basic Barbecue Sauce

You can store this barbecue sauce in your refrigerator up to 2 weeks. It's great to have on hand as a dipping sauce for your Turnip Fries (Chapter 7) or to pour over your burgers.

INGREDIENTS | SERVES 6

2 (6-ounce) cans tomato paste

½ cup apple cider vinegar

⅓ cup granulated erythritol

2 teaspoons smoked paprika

¾ teaspoon garlic powder

¾ teaspoon onion powder

½ teaspoon salt

¼ teaspoon chili powder

⅛ teaspoon cayenne pepper

1 cup water

1. Add all ingredients to a medium saucepan and whisk over medium-high heat. Allow mixture to come to a slight boil, then reduce heat to low.

2. Allow to simmer 20 minutes or until mixture starts to thicken.

3. If sauce is thicker than you like, you can stir in more water. Otherwise, remove from heat and allow to cool. Store in an airtight container in the refrigerator.

PER SERVING Calories: 54 | Fat: 0 g | Protein: 3 g | Sodium: 638 mg | Fiber: 2.5 g | Carbohydrates: 18 g | Sugar: 7 g

Ketchup

Simmering this ketchup for a few minutes helps develop the flavors a little more, but if you want to save time, you can skip this step and just mix everything together before transferring to an airtight container. This ketchup will keep in the refrigerator up to 2 weeks.

INGREDIENTS | SERVES 6

6 ounces tomato paste

2 tablespoons apple cider vinegar

⅔ cup water

¼ teaspoon garlic powder

¼ teaspoon onion powder

⅛ teaspoon ground cloves

⅛ teaspoon allspice

2 drops liquid stevia

¾ teaspoon salt

1. Combine all ingredients in a medium saucepan over low heat.

2. Stir until combined and bring to a simmer. Allow to simmer 3 minutes.

3. Remove from heat and allow to cool. Once cooled, transfer to an airtight container and store in the refrigerator.

PER SERVING   Calories: 24 | Fat: 0 g | Protein: 1 g | Sodium: 513 mg | Fiber: 2.5 g | Carbohydrates: 6 g | Sugar: 4 g

Nacho Cheese Sauce

This cheese sauce may look hardened and clumpy when stored in the refrigerator over the course of the week, but it will smooth out when you heat it back up. It makes a great addition to the Cheesy Cauliflower Tots (Chapter 10). You can store this Nacho Cheese Sauce in the refrigerator up to 1 week.

INGREDIENTS | SERVES 6

4 ounces cream cheese

4 tablespoons full-fat coconut milk

2 tablespoons ghee

2 ounces grated white Cheddar cheese

½ teaspoon paprika

½ teaspoon Worcestershire sauce

1. Combine all ingredients in a medium saucepan over medium heat.

2. Stir until everything is melted and incorporated.

3. Store in an airtight container in the refrigerator.

PER SERVING   Calories: 158 | Fat: 15 g | Protein: 4 g | Sodium: 134 mg | Fiber: 0 g | Carbohydrates: 2 g | Sugar: 0.5 g

Worcestershire's Main Ingredient

Worcestershire sauce is made from anchovies that have been fermented in vinegar for eighteen months. The flavor of Worcestershire sauce, which is referred to as umami, is hard to replicate with any other sauce.

Enchilada Sauce

You can store this enchilada sauce in your refrigerator for about a week and a half. It's used in several recipes, so you can get a head start by making this sauce in advance and using it straight from the refrigerator when cooking.

INGREDIENTS | SERVES 6

2 cups no-sugar-added chicken broth
2 tablespoons tomato paste
3 tablespoons chili powder
1½ teaspoons ground cumin
¾ teaspoon dried oregano
½ teaspoon salt
½ teaspoon onion powder
½ teaspoon garlic powder
½ teaspoon granulated erythritol
⅛ teaspoon ground clove
⅛ teaspoon ground cinnamon
2 tablespoons ghee
½ teaspoon arrowroot powder

1. Combine all ingredients in a medium saucepan over medium heat.

2. Bring to a simmer and allow to cook, stirring occasionally, until sauce is reduced by about ⅓ and thickened, about 6 minutes.

3. Transfer to an airtight container.

PER SERVING Calories: 70 | Fat: 5 g | Protein: 3 g | Sodium: 378 mg | Fiber: 2 g | Carbohydrates: 5 g | Sugar: 1 g

Alfredo Sauce

Full-fat coconut milk only lasts about 1 week in the refrigerator. If you want to make this sauce further in advance and you can tolerate dairy, you can make it with cream instead of coconut milk and store it up to 2 weeks.

INGREDIENTS | SERVES 6

6 tablespoons ghee
1 cup full-fat coconut milk
⅛ teaspoon ground nutmeg
⅛ teaspoon salt
¼ cup grated Parmesan cheese

1. Melt ghee in a small saucepan over low heat, being careful not to let it boil.

2. Whisk coconut milk into melted ghee and allow to simmer 1–2 minutes.

3. Remove from heat and add remaining ingredients. Stir until smooth.

4. Store in an airtight container in the refrigerator.

PER SERVING Calories: 204 | Fat: 21 g | Protein: 2 g | Sodium: 128 mg | Fiber: 0 g | Carbohydrates: 2 g | Sugar: 0 g

Creamy Garlic Dip

This dip is excellent to have on hand as a side for low-carb sliced vegetables. You can store it in small dressing containers inside a larger container with cut-up cucumbers and peppers in the refrigerator up to 1 week for a quick, nutritious snack on the go.

INGREDIENTS | SERVES 6

¾ cup Basic Mayonnaise (see recipe in this chapter)

2 drops liquid stevia

4 cloves garlic, minced

1½ tablespoons olive oil

1 tablespoon white vinegar

⅓ teaspoon lemon juice

2 teaspoons fish sauce

1. Combine all ingredients in a small bowl and whisk until incorporated.

2. Store in an airtight container in the refrigerator.

PER SERVING Calories: 232 | Fat: 25 g | Protein: 1 g | Sodium: 205 mg | Fiber: 0 g | Carbohydrates: 2 g | Sugar: 0 g

Chipotle Peppers in Adobo Sauce

Canned varieties of chipotle peppers often contain sugar, high-fructose corn syrup, and flour—three ingredients that don't mesh well with a low-carb diet. The good news is it's easy to make your own, and they last in the refrigerator up to 3 weeks as long as they are sealed tightly.

INGREDIENTS | SERVES 10

10 dried chipotle chilies, stemmed and slit lengthwise

⅓ cup sliced white onion

5 tablespoons apple cider vinegar

2 cloves garlic, thinly sliced

4 tablespoons no-sugar-added tomato sauce

½ teaspoon cumin

¼ teaspoon salt

¼ teaspoon cinnamon

⅛ teaspoon allspice

3 cups water

1. Combine all ingredients in a medium saucepan and cook covered over low heat for 1 hour. Uncover and continue cooking 30 minutes, allowing liquid to reduce to around 1 cup.

2. Remove from heat and transfer to an airtight container. Store in the refrigerator.

PER SERVING Calories: 24 | Fat: 0 g | Protein: 1 g | Sodium: 92 mg | Fiber: 1 g | Carbohydrates: 5 g | Sugar: 2 g

CHAPTER 10

Sides

Cauliflower Mash

The key to making this dish super creamy is the food processor. You can make it with a potato masher or an immersion blender, too, but you won't get the same mashed potato–like texture that you would in a food processor. This will keep in the refrigerator up to 1 week.

INGREDIENTS | SERVES 6

3 cups water

1 large head of cauliflower, cut into florets

2 tablespoons ghee

¼ cup no-sugar-added chicken broth

1 teaspoon salt

½ teaspoon freshly ground black pepper

1. Fill a large pot with water. Bring to a boil. Add cauliflower and cook until softened, about 7 minutes.

2. Strain cauliflower and transfer to a food processor. Process until cauliflower is broken up into fine chunks.

3. Stop food processor and add ghee. Turn food processor back on to low and slowly add chicken broth while food processor is running. Add more liquid if necessary to get desired consistency.

4. Once cauliflower is smooth, add salt and pepper and process until combined.

5. Divide evenly among six airtight containers and store in the refrigerator until ready to eat.

PER SERVING Calories: 63 | Fat: 4 g | Protein: 2 g | Sodium: 420 mg | Fiber: 2 g | Carbohydrates: 5 g | Sugar: 2 g

Zucchini Tots

These zucchini tots are delicious hot or cold. If you want to heat them up, add a little oil to a medium pan over medium heat and cook them 2 minutes, gently stirring until heated through. Serve with ketchup or your favorite dipping sauce. These tots will keep in the refrigerator for up to 1 week.

INGREDIENTS | SERVES 6 (MAKES 30 TOTS)

2 cups shredded zucchini
1 cup coarsely ground almond flour
1½ teaspoons Italian seasoning
½ cup shredded Parmesan cheese
1 jumbo egg (or 1 whole large egg and 1 large egg white)

Egg Sizes

Eggs typically come in four sizes: jumbo, extra large, large, and medium. Large is the most common size used in recipes and the most readily available, but most grocery stores also sell jumbo eggs.

1. Preheat oven to 400°F. Line a baking sheet with parchment paper.

2. After shredding zucchini, use a paper towel to pat it dry. Zucchini won't be completely dry, but remove as much excess moisture as you can.

3. Add all ingredients to a large mixing bowl and stir until everything is combined.

4. Take about 1 tablespoon of the mixture in your hand and form into a cylindrical tater tot shape. Place on lined baking sheet. Repeat until all mixture is formed into tots.

5. Bake 17 minutes or until bottom is slightly browned. Flip tots over and bake another 5 minutes.

6. Divide evenly among six airtight containers and store in the refrigerator until ready to eat.

PER SERVING Calories: 107 | Fat: 2 g | Protein: 5 g | Sodium: 51 mg | Fiber: 1 g | Carbohydrates: 17 g | Sugar: 1 g

Coconut Curry Roasted Cauliflower

This roasted cauliflower is a meal prep staple. It's quick and inexpensive, and it makes a great side dish for most proteins—steak, chicken, and pork. You can adjust seasonings to your liking or experiment with different combinations to switch things up during your meal prep. It will keep in the refrigerator 1 week.

INGREDIENTS | SERVES 6

1 large head of cauliflower, cut into bite-sized florets

1 heaping tablespoon coconut oil, melted

1½ teaspoons curry powder

1 teaspoon salt

½ teaspoon freshly ground black pepper

2 teaspoons lemon juice

1. Preheat oven to 425°F.

2. Combine cauliflower and coconut oil in a medium bowl and toss to coat. Add spices and toss again to make sure cauliflower is evenly coated.

3. Spread cauliflower out in a single layer on a baking sheet. Roast 10 minutes or until bottom of cauliflower starts to brown. Flip each piece over and roast another 5 minutes.

4. Transfer roasted cauliflower to a medium bowl and toss with lemon juice.

5. Store in an airtight container in the refrigerator until ready to eat.

PER SERVING Calories: 46 | Fat: 3 g | Protein: 2 g | Sodium: 417 mg | Fiber: 2 g | Carbohydrates: 5 g | Sugar: 2 g

Roasted Green Beans and Mushrooms

This is a basic side dish that pairs well with any of the poultry, beef, or pork entrées that don't have a vegetable component. These will last in the refrigerator up to 1 week.

INGREDIENTS | SERVES 6

¼ cup olive oil

2 tablespoons coconut aminos

2 cloves garlic, minced

1 teaspoon salt

1 teaspoon freshly ground black pepper

2 cups green beans

1 cup sliced white mushrooms

1. Preheat oven to 400°F.

2. Combine olive oil, coconut aminos, garlic, salt, and pepper in a medium mixing bowl.

3. Add green beans and mushrooms and toss to combine.

4. Spread out on a baking sheet and bake 20–25 minutes or until green beans are tender.

5. Divide into six equal portions and store each portion in a separate airtight container in the refrigerator until ready to eat.

PER SERVING Calories: 104 | Fat: 9 g | Protein: 2 g | Sodium: 535 mg | Fiber: 2 g | Carbohydrates: 5 g | Sugar: 2 g

Garlic Roasted Mushrooms

White mushrooms tend to have the mildest mushroom flavor, so they go well with any protein dish, but you can use your favorite kind of mushroom in this recipe with the same great results. Keep these in the refrigerator up to 1 week.

INGREDIENTS | SERVES 6

1 pound white mushrooms, cut in half

2 cloves garlic, minced

2 tablespoons olive oil

2 teaspoons lemon juice

¼ cup chopped cilantro

½ teaspoon salt

½ teaspoon freshly ground black pepper

2 tablespoons ghee

Soapy Cilantro?

To between 4 and 14 percent of the population, cilantro tastes just like soap. Research has concluded that these people all share a similar genetic trait that affects olfactory-receptor genes (the genes that affect your sense of smell). People with this genetic trait are able to pick up on the smell of aldehyde chemicals, which are found in both cilantro and soap.

1. Preheat oven to 450°F. Spray a 9" × 9" baking dish with nonstick cooking spray.

2. Add mushrooms, garlic, olive oil, lemon juice, cilantro, salt, and pepper to dish and toss to coat mushrooms.

3. Spread mushrooms out and evenly dot the top with ghee.

4. Roast 10 minutes, stir, and then continue roasting another 10 minutes.

5. Divide into six equal portions and store each portion in a separate airtight container in the refrigerator until ready to eat.

PER SERVING   Calories: 95 | Fat: 9 g | Protein: 2.5 g | Sodium: 198 mg | Fiber: 1 g | Carbohydrates: 3 g | Sugar: 1.5 g

Cheesy Cauliflower Tots

These tots are the perfect complement to any protein dish. They also pair well with scrambled eggs. They'll last in the refrigerator up to 1 week. The best way to heat them up is by adding a little ghee to a medium pan and heating for a few minutes over medium heat.

INGREDIENTS | SERVES 6 (MAKES 30 TOTS)

1 cup water

2 cups cauliflower florets

1 large egg

½ cup minced onion

¼ cup shredded Cheddar cheese

¼ cup grated Parmesan cheese

¼ cup coarsely ground almond flour

2 tablespoons minced fresh parsley

½ teaspoon salt

¼ teaspoon freshly ground black pepper

1. Preheat oven to 375°F. Spray a baking sheet with nonstick cooking spray.

2. Combine water and cauliflower in a medium pot and heat over medium heat. Allow to come to a boil and then reduce heat to low and cover. Steam cauliflower 3–5 minutes or until fork tender.

3. Drain cauliflower and then transfer to a food processor and pulse until cauliflower is broken up into fine pieces.

4. Combine all ingredients in a medium mixing bowl and stir until incorporated. Use your hands to shape about a tablespoon of cauliflower mixture into a cylindrical tot shape. Place on baking sheet. Repeat until mixture is gone.

5. Bake 10 minutes, flip tots over, and then bake another 10 minutes or until golden brown.

6. Store in an airtight container in the refrigerator until ready to eat.

PER SERVING   Calories: 85 | Fat: 4 g | Protein: 5 g | Sodium: 328 mg | Fiber: 1 g | Carbohydrates: 8 g | Sugar: 1 g

Roasted Cauliflower

Because this cauliflower is roasted whole, this side dish comes together quickly. If you prefer, you can cut the cauliflower into florets before roasting and mix everything in a large bowl, roasting on a baking sheet. This dish will last in the refrigerator up to 1 week.

INGREDIENTS | SERVES 6

1 large head cauliflower
6 heaping tablespoons ghee, softened
¼ teaspoon dry mustard powder
2 cloves garlic, minced
1 tablespoon dried dill

What's the Deal with Dry Mustard?

Dry mustard powder is the dried version of prepared mustard. To make mustard, dry mustard powder is mixed with spices, herbs, and liquid—typically a mixture of water and vinegar. In most cases you can substitute prepared mustard for dry mustard powder in the ratio of 3 to 1. For example, if a recipe calls for 1 teaspoon of dry mustard powder, you can use 1 tablespoon of prepared mustard instead.

1. Preheat oven to 350°F.

2. Cut stem off cauliflower so that cauliflower has a flat bottom and stands evenly. Place cauliflower in an 8" × 8" baking dish.

3. In a small bowl, combine ghee, mustard powder, garlic, and dill. Spread ghee mixture over entire cauliflower, making sure to cover evenly. Cover dish with foil.

4. Roast 75 minutes or until cauliflower is tender throughout. Remove from oven and use a spoon to pour any excess liquid over top of cauliflower.

5. Allow to cool, then cut into six equal portions for meal prepping.

6. Store in an airtight container in the refrigerator until ready to eat.

PER SERVING Calories: 138 | Fat: 13 g | Protein: 2 g | Sodium: 32 mg | Fiber: 2 g | Carbohydrates: 5 g | Sugar: 1.5 g

Parmesan Zucchini Bites

You can quickly reheat these bites by adding a little olive oil to a medium pan over medium heat. Once olive oil is hot, add zucchini bites and heat 1 minute, flip, then heat 1 more minute. These bites will last up to 1 week in the refrigerator.

INGREDIENTS | SERVES 6

1 large egg
1 large egg white
1 cup Parmesan cheese
¼ cup chopped fresh parsley
½ teaspoon garlic powder
¼ teaspoon onion powder
2 large zucchini, cut into rounds

1. Preheat oven to 425°F. Spray two baking sheets with nonstick cooking spray or line with parchment paper.

2. Whisk egg and egg white together in a small bowl.

3. In a separate small bowl, combine Parmesan cheese, parsley, garlic powder, and onion powder.

4. Dip each zucchini slice in egg and then into Parmesan mixture and fully coat. Place zucchini slice on baking sheet and repeat with all remaining slices, arranging zucchini in a single layer.

5. Bake 10 minutes, flip slices over, and then bake 10 minutes more or until golden brown. Remove from oven and allow to cool slightly.

6. Divide into 6 equal portions and store each portion in a separate airtight container in the refrigerator until ready to eat.

PER SERVING   Calories: 52 | Fat: 2 g | Protein: 5 g | Sodium: 96 mg | Fiber: 1 g | Carbohydrates: 4 g | Sugar: 3 g

Spicy Broccoli

If you want to make this broccoli even spicier, you can add a dash or two of hot sauce right after the broccoli comes out of the oven or right before eating. You can keep this broccoli in the refrigerator up to 1 week.

INGREDIENTS | SERVES 6

1 cup water
4 cups bite-sized broccoli florets
¼ cup Basic Mayonnaise (Chapter 9)
2 teaspoons sriracha
1 teaspoon coconut aminos

Steaming versus Boiling

Steaming broccoli helps preserve more nutrients than boiling. Water-soluble vitamins, which include the B vitamins and vitamin C, are destroyed by both water and heat, so when you boil broccoli, a lot of these nutrients are lost. It's best to cook broccoli by steaming or roasting for as little time as possible.

1. Turn oven on to broil.

2. Put water in the bottom pot of a double boiler and broccoli in the top pot. Turn to medium heat and allow broccoli to steam 6 minutes or until bright green yet still crunchy.

3. In a medium bowl, combine mayonnaise, sriracha, and coconut aminos. Add broccoli and toss to coat.

4. Transfer coated broccoli to a baking sheet and broil 3 minutes. Flip broccoli and broil 3 more minutes or until slightly browned. Divide into six equal portions and store each portion in a separate airtight container in the refrigerator until ready to eat.

PER SERVING Calories: 87 | Fat: 7 g | Protein: 2 g | Sodium: 196 mg | Fiber: 2 g | Carbohydrates: 4 g | Sugar: 1 g

Garlic Roasted Asparagus

You can easily change this recipe if you want some variety. Add a little Parmesan cheese or some red pepper flakes or throw in some mushrooms with the asparagus. You can keep this in the refrigerator up to 1 week.

INGREDIENTS | SERVES 6

4 tablespoons olive oil
1 teaspoon salt
3 cloves garlic, minced
1 bunch asparagus, trimmed
2 tablespoons lemon juice

1. Preheat oven to 425°F.

2. Combine olive oil, salt, and garlic in a medium mixing bowl. Add asparagus and toss until it is evenly coated.

3. Roast asparagus 10 minutes or until tender.

4. Remove from oven, return to bowl, add lemon juice, and toss to coat.

5. Divide into six equal portions and store each portion in a separate airtight container in the refrigerator until ready to eat.

PER SERVING Calories: 89 | Fat: 9 g | Protein: 1 g | Sodium: 388 mg | Fiber: 1 g | Carbohydrates: 2 g | Sugar: 1 g

Spicy Creamed Spinach

The arrowroot powder in this recipe will cause it to thicken up a bit as it sits in the refrigerator over the course of the week. If you want to thin it out, just add a teaspoon or so of coconut milk to your serving before heating it back up. Store in the refrigerator up to 1 week.

INGREDIENTS | SERVES 6

¼ cup coconut milk

⅛ teaspoon arrowroot powder

¼ teaspoon crushed red pepper flakes

¼ teaspoon salt

4 cups baby spinach

1. Heat coconut milk in a medium saucepan over medium heat. When coconut milk is hot but not boiling, add arrowroot powder and stir until milk starts to thicken.

2. Add red pepper flakes and salt and stir to combine. Stir in spinach and cook until wilted, about 2 minutes.

3. Divide into six equal portions and store each portion in a separate airtight container in the refrigerator until ready to eat.

PER SERVING Calories: 23 | Fat: 2 g | Protein: 1 g | Sodium: 113 mg | Fiber: 0.5 g | Carbohydrates: 1 g | Sugar: 0 g

Salt and Vinegar Radish Chips

Radishes are little, but they pack a big crunch. If you prefer, you can eat your radishes raw. Follow the directions as written, but skip the cooking! They'll soften a bit in the vinegar, but they'll still be delicious. Either way, these chips will last in the refrigerator up to 1 week.

INGREDIENTS | SERVES 6

2 tablespoons olive oil

1 tablespoon apple cider vinegar

1 pound fresh radishes, sliced thinly, using a mandoline if possible

½ teaspoon salt

½ teaspoon freshly ground black pepper

1. Preheat oven to 400°F. Line two baking sheets with parchment paper.

2. Whisk together olive oil and vinegar in a medium mixing bowl. Add radishes and toss to coat.

3. Arrange radish slices in a single layer on baking sheets. Sprinkle salt and pepper over slices.

4. Bake 15 minutes and remove from oven.

5. Divide into six equal portions and store each portion in a separate airtight container in the refrigerator until ready to eat.

PER SERVING Calories: 52 | Fat: 4 g | Protein: 0.5 g | Sodium: 223 mg | Fiber: 1 g | Carbohydrates: 2.5 g | Sugar: 1 g

Mozzarella and Basil Tomatoes

These are superb chilled, but if you want to warm them up a little before eating, put them under the broiler for 2–3 minutes or quickly heat them up in the toaster oven. Store in the refrigerator up to 1 week.

INGREDIENTS | SERVES 6 (MAKES 12 TOMATO SLICES)

6 medium Roma tomatoes, ends sliced off and cut in half crosswise
½ teaspoon salt
½ teaspoon garlic powder
½ teaspoon onion powder
½ teaspoon Italian seasoning
½ teaspoon dried parsley
¼ teaspoon freshly ground black pepper
12 fresh basil leaves
½ cup shredded mozzarella cheese

1. Preheat oven to 425°F. Line a baking sheet with parchment paper.

2. Arrange cut tomatoes on baking sheet.

3. Combine spices and seasonings in a small bowl. Sprinkle on tomato slices, flip slices over, and sprinkle on the other side.

4. Place a basil leaf on each tomato and sprinkle cheese on top.

5. Bake 15–20 minutes or until cheese is slightly golden and tomatoes are tender. Divide into six equal portions and store each portion in a separate airtight container in the refrigerator until ready to eat.

PER SERVING Calories: 39 | Fat: 2 g | Protein: 3 g | Sodium: 255 mg | Fiber: 1 g | Carbohydrates: 2.5 g | Sugar: 1 g

Spicy Sugar Snap Peas

Sugar snap peas have a string on each side of their pods that should be removed before cooking. To prepare sugar snap peas properly, snap the stem end and pull off the string on both sides. You can store these sugar snap peas in the refrigerator up to 1 week.

INGREDIENTS | SERVES 6

2 tablespoons coconut aminos

1 teaspoon sesame oil

1 teaspoon sriracha

⅛ teaspoon ground ginger

2 tablespoons avocado oil

1½ pounds sugar snap peas, sliced lengthwise

2 teaspoons sesame seeds

1. In a medium mixing bowl, combine coconut aminos, sesame oil, sriracha, and ginger. Whisk until combined.

2. Heat avocado oil in a medium skillet over high heat. Add peas and cook until peas turn bright green, about 3 minutes. Transfer peas to bowl with sesame oil mixture and toss to coat. Sprinkle sesame seeds on top and toss again.

3. Divide into six equal portions and store each portion in a separate airtight container in the refrigerator until ready to eat.

PER SERVING Calories: 104 | Fat: 6 g | Protein: 4 g | Sodium: 179 mg | Fiber: 3 g | Carbohydrates: 9 g | Sugar: 4 g

Sesame Broccoli with Red Peppers

If you want to make this a full meal, you can add some ground beef or turkey to the skillet after cooking the vegetables and cook until it's no longer pink. Then just divide into portions, store in the refrigerator, and you're set for six meals during the week.

INGREDIENTS | SERVES 6

2 tablespoons sesame oil

3 cups chopped broccoli

½ medium green bell pepper, seeded and sliced

½ medium red bell pepper, seeded and sliced

½ medium yellow bell pepper, seeded and sliced

2 tablespoons coconut aminos

2 tablespoons sesame seeds

1. Heat sesame oil in a medium skillet over medium-high heat. Add broccoli and cook until it starts to soften, about 3 minutes. Add peppers and cook 3 more minutes. Stir in coconut aminos, making sure vegetables are coated.

2. Remove from heat and toss vegetables with sesame seeds.

3. Divide into six equal portions and store each portion in a separate airtight container in the refrigerator until ready to eat.

PER SERVING Calories: 84 | Fat: 6 g | Protein: 2 g | Sodium: 160 mg | Fiber: 2 g | Carbohydrates: 6 g | Sugar: 2 g

Roasted Celery Root and Radishes

Celery root has a texture similar to that of potatoes with less than half the carbohydrates. A half cup of celery root contains only 7 grams of carbohydrates, while a cup of potatoes contains around 16 grams. This dish will keep up to 1 week in the refrigerator.

INGREDIENTS | SERVES 6

3 tablespoons olive oil

½ teaspoon salt

½ teaspoon freshly ground black pepper

½ teaspoon dried thyme

¼ teaspoon garlic powder

1 pound celery root, peeled and cubed

1 pound radishes, cubed

Celery Root by Any Other Name

Celery root is also called celeriac, turnip-rooted celery, or knob celery. When choosing celery root, look for unblemished skin that has a greenish hue. To prepare celery root, scrub it well, cut off the top and bottom, and peel off the skin with a vegetable peeler.

1. Preheat oven to 325°F.

2. Whisk olive oil, salt, pepper, thyme, and garlic powder together in a large bowl.

3. Add celery root and radishes and toss to coat.

4. Spread celery root and radishes out on a baking sheet and bake 25 minutes or until tender and slightly browned.

5. Divide into six equal portions and store each portion in a separate airtight container in the refrigerator until ready to eat.

PER SERVING   Calories: 104 | Fat: 7 g | Protein: 2 g | Sodium: 297 mg | Fiber: 3 g | Carbohydrates: 9 g | Sugar: 2 g

Fried Swiss Chard

To reheat this Swiss chard, heat ghee in a medium skillet over medium-high heat. Add chard and quickly sauté 1–2 minutes until just heated through. This will keep in the refrigerator up to 1 week.

INGREDIENTS | SERVES 6

6 slices no-sugar-added bacon, chopped

3 tablespoons ghee

3 cloves garlic, minced

4 tablespoons fresh lemon juice

2 bunches Swiss chard, stems removed and finely chopped

1 teaspoon salt

½ teaspoon freshly ground black pepper

Chard, the Vitamin K Powerhouse

Just 1 cup of Swiss chard provides over three times the amount of vitamin K you need for the entire day. Swiss chard also contains natural nitrates, which have been shown to lower blood pressure and help improve athletic performance.

1. Heat a large skillet over medium heat. Add chopped bacon and cook until bacon turns crisp, about 5 minutes.

2. Add ghee to skillet. Once it melts, add garlic and lemon juice and stir, cooking 1 minute. Add Swiss chard, stir to coat, and cover.

3. Allow chard to cook 5 minutes covered. Stir chard, testing for doneness. If needed, cook 2 more minutes. Stir in salt and pepper.

4. Remove from heat. Divide into six equal portions and store each portion in a separate airtight container in the refrigerator until ready to eat.

PER SERVING Calories: 179 | Fat: 17 g | Protein: 4 g | Sodium: 601 mg | Fiber: 2 g | Carbohydrates: 2 g | Sugar: 0.5 g

Fried Cabbage

This goes really well with pork as a main dish. When planning your meals for the week, you may want to consider pairing this side with the Roasted Pork Loin. Just portion the pork out, add a serving of fried cabbage to the same container, and store in the refrigerator up to 1 week.

INGREDIENTS | SERVES 6

2 tablespoons ghee

1½ cups chopped celery

6 cups shredded green cabbage

1½ cups diced red bell pepper

½ cup minced yellow onion

1 tablespoon coconut aminos

⅛ teaspoon freshly ground black pepper

1. Heat ghee in medium skillet over medium heat. Add celery and cook until starting to soften, about 2 minutes. Add cabbage, bell pepper, and onion, and continue to cook until vegetables start to become tender but still have some crispness, about 4 minutes.

2. Add coconut aminos and black pepper and stir to combine. Remove from heat.

3. Divide into six equal portions and store each portion in a separate airtight container in the refrigerator until ready to eat.

PER SERVING   Calories: 83 | Fat: 4 g | Protein: 2 g | Sodium: 114 mg | Fiber: 4 g | Carbohydrates: 9 g | Sugar: 5 g

Mashed Turnips

These turnips may thicken as they sit in the refrigerator during the week. If you want to thin them out, you can add a bit more almond milk or some coconut milk right before heating. Stir the milk in once the turnips are warmed up, and they'll be back to their original texture.

INGREDIENTS | SERVES 6

6 cups water
5 large turnips, peeled and cubed
3 tablespoons ghee
2 shallots, minced
1 tablespoon dried sage
1 cup unsweetened almond milk
1 teaspoon salt
½ teaspoon freshly ground black pepper
1 teaspoon dried chives

1. Add water and turnips to a large stockpot. Bring to a boil over high heat, then reduce heat and allow to simmer until softened, about 20 minutes.

2. While turnips are cooking, melt ghee in a small saucepan over medium heat. Add shallots and sage and sauté until shallots soften, about 3 minutes. Add almond milk and allow to simmer.

3. Drain turnips and put back into pot. Add almond milk mixture and use an immersion blender or handheld electric mixer to beat until smooth. Stir in salt, pepper, and chives.

4. Divide into six equal portions and store each portion in a separate airtight container in the refrigerator until ready to eat.

PER SERVING Calories: 121 | Fat: 7 g | Protein: 2.5 g | Sodium: 510 mg | Fiber: 3 g | Carbohydrates: 12 g | Sugar: 7 g

Green Bean Casserole

Green bean casserole is a Thanksgiving favorite, but this low-carb version is great for meal prep too. The addition of cream cheese makes it creamy, so it holds up well in the refrigerator up to 1 week.

INGREDIENTS | SERVES 6

1 pound green beans, trimmed

8 ounces cream cheese

1 cup full-fat coconut milk

1 cup almond milk

1 teaspoon garlic powder

½ teaspoon salt

¼ cup grated Parmesan cheese

¾ cup shredded mozzarella cheese

Get Regular with Green Beans

Green beans are exceptionally rich in fiber, which keeps digestion regular, helps you lose weight, and can contribute to a healthy blood sugar level. One cup of green beans contains 3.5 grams of fiber, almost 15 percent of the amount you need for the entire day.

1. Preheat oven to 350°F.

2. Steam green beans in a double boiler until softened, about 8 minutes.

3. While green beans steam, combine all remaining ingredients except mozzarella cheese in a small saucepan. Stir until smooth.

4. Transfer cooked green beans to a 9" × 13" baking dish and pour cream cheese mixture on top. Stir to coat.

5. Sprinkle mozzarella cheese on top and cook 25 minutes or until cheese is bubbly and browned.

6. Divide into six equal portions and store each portion in a separate airtight container. Store in the refrigerator until ready to eat.

PER SERVING   Calories: 308 | Fat: 26 g | Protein: 10 g | Sodium: 534 mg | Fiber: 2 g | Carbohydrates: 11 g | Sugar: 5 g

CHAPTER 11

Soups

Chicken Zoodle Soup

This low-carb soup is even better for meal prep than the classic chicken noodle soup because the zucchini is already so naturally moisture rich that it doesn't soak up all the broth in the soup as it sits. This soup will last up to 1 week in the refrigerator.

INGREDIENTS | SERVES 6

2 tablespoons olive oil, divided

1 pound boneless, skinless chicken breasts, cut into 1" cubes

1½ teaspoons salt, divided

1 teaspoon freshly ground black pepper, divided

2 cloves garlic, minced

1 medium yellow onion, peeled and diced

3 stalks celery, chopped

5 cups no-sugar-added chicken broth

½ teaspoon dried thyme

½ teaspoon dried rosemary

2 bay leaves

2 tablespoons chopped fresh parsley

1 tablespoon lemon juice

3 large zucchini, spiralized

1. Heat 1 tablespoon olive oil in a large stockpot over medium heat. Add chicken and season with ¾ teaspoon salt and ½ teaspoon pepper. Cook chicken until browned, about 3 minutes on each side.

2. Remove chicken and set aside.

3. Add remaining olive oil to stockpot along with garlic, onion, and celery. Cook until tender, about 4 minutes, stirring occasionally.

4. Add chicken broth, thyme, rosemary, bay leaves, parsley, lemon juice, and remaining salt and pepper and bring to a boil over high heat. Stir in zucchini noodles and chicken and reduce heat to low. Cook until zucchini is tender, about 4 minutes.

5. Remove from heat and allow to cool.

6. Divide evenly among six airtight containers. Store in the refrigerator until ready to eat.

PER SERVING Calories: 205 | Fat: 8 g | Protein: 23 g | Sodium: 715 mg | Fiber: 3 g | Carbohydrates: 11 g | Sugar: 5.5 g

Cream of Mushroom Soup

This soup calls for coconut milk, which tends to be thicker than almond milk, but if you prefer, you can substitute almond milk in the same ratio. You can store this soup in the refrigerator up to 1 week.

INGREDIENTS | SERVES 6

6 cups cauliflower florets

3 cups coconut milk

2 cups no-sugar-added chicken broth

2 teaspoons onion powder

1 teaspoon garlic powder

1 teaspoon salt

½ teaspoon freshly ground black pepper

2 teaspoons olive oil

4 cups diced white mushrooms

1 large yellow onion, peeled and diced

Fibrous Mushrooms

Mushrooms have two types of dietary fiber in their cell walls—beta glucans and chitin. Both these fibers pull water into the digestive tract, helping to make you feel fuller faster and longer and reducing appetite over the long term. Because fiber doesn't count toward your net carbohydrates, mushrooms are a great addition to a low-carbohydrate diet.

1. Combine cauliflower, coconut milk, chicken broth, onion powder, garlic powder, salt, and pepper in a large stockpot. Cover and bring to a boil over medium-high heat. Once mixture starts to boil, reduce heat to low and allow to simmer until cauliflower is tender, about 7 minutes.

2. Use an immersion blender to purée mixture. Set aside.

3. Heat olive oil in a medium skillet over medium heat. Add mushrooms and onion and cook until mushrooms are softened, 4–5 minutes. Transfer half the mushroom mixture to the cauliflower mixture and purée with immersion blender.

4. Add remaining mushrooms and onions and stir until combined.

5. Divide evenly among six airtight containers. Store in the refrigerator until ready to eat.

PER SERVING Calories: 319 | Fat: 26 g | Protein: 9 g | Sodium: 462 mg | Fiber: 5 g | Carbohydrates: 18 g | Sugar: 5 g

Buffalo Chicken Soup

This recipe calls for shredded canned chicken because it's already ready to go and can save you even more time while you're meal prepping; however, if you prefer, you can prepare your own shredded chicken and use it in place of the canned chicken. This soup will keep all week in the refrigerator.

INGREDIENTS | SERVES 6

2 tablespoons ghee

¼ cup chopped yellow onion

3 stalks celery, chopped

1 teaspoon salt

½ teaspoon freshly ground black pepper

1 tablespoon tomato paste

3 cups no-sugar-added chicken broth

¼ cup Frank's RedHot

4 ounces cream cheese, softened

1 cup full-fat coconut milk

3 cups shredded canned chicken

1. Heat ghee in a large stockpot over medium heat. Add onion and celery and cook until softened, about 4 minutes.

2. Add salt, pepper, and tomato paste and stir until combined. Add chicken broth and hot sauce. Bring to a boil and then reduce heat to low and allow to simmer.

3. Add cream cheese and stir until melted and fully incorporated. Stir in coconut milk and shredded chicken.

4. Divide evenly among six airtight containers. Store in the refrigerator until ready to eat.

PER SERVING Calories: 395 | Fat: 27 g | Protein: 30 g | Sodium: 1,038 mg | Fiber: 1 g | Carbohydrates: 6 g | Sugar: 2 g

Cream of Tomato Soup

The macadamia nuts in this soup add a creaminess that's hard to achieve with other types of nuts. If you can, make the recipe as is instead of substituting something else. It's worth it! This soup will keep up to 1 week in the refrigerator.

INGREDIENTS | SERVES 6

6 large vine-ripened tomatoes, chopped and seeded

¾ cup sun-dried tomatoes

¾ cup raw macadamia nuts

1 teaspoon salt

½ teaspoon freshly ground black pepper

¼ cup fresh basil

2 cloves garlic

5 cups vegetable broth, warmed

1 cup unsweetened almond milk, warmed

1. Combine all ingredients in a high-powered blender. Blend until smooth and heated through, about 5 minutes.

2. Divide evenly among six airtight containers. Store in the refrigerator until ready to eat.

PER SERVING Calories: 230 | Fat: 13 g | Protein: 5 g | Sodium: 535 mg | Fiber: 5 g | Carbohydrates: 16 g | Sugar: 9 g

Smoked Chicken Chowder

It's important to use the full-fat coconut milk for this recipe to get the chowder feel. The coconut milk you find in the carton is not as thick. Many boxed coconut milks also contain a lot of undesirable ingredients, while coconut milk in the can is only one or two ingredients. This chowder can last in the refrigerator up to 1 week.

INGREDIENTS | SERVES 6

6 slices no-sugar-added bacon, diced

1 medium yellow onion, peeled and chopped

4 cups cubed jicama

2 cloves garlic, minced

1 pound boneless, skinless chicken breasts, cut into 1" cubes

3 cups no-sugar-added chicken broth

1 teaspoon salt

½ teaspoon freshly ground black pepper

2 cups full-fat coconut milk

1 teaspoon arrowroot powder

1 chipotle pepper in adobo sauce, minced

Chipotles in Adobo Sauce

Chipotles in adobo sauce give this smoked chowder its signature spicy, smoked flavor. Although most canned chipotles in adobo sauce do contain some sugar, they are still considered low-carb. That being said, it's best to avoid white sugar as much as possible, so if time allows, make your own chipotles in adobo sauce.

1. Cook bacon until crispy in a large stockpot over medium heat. When bacon is cooked, transfer to a plate lined with a paper towel.

2. Add onion and jicama to bacon grease in stockpot and cook until tender, about 8 minutes. Add garlic and cook 1 more minute. Add chicken and cook until no longer pink and juices run clear, about 7 minutes.

3. Add remaining ingredients and bring to a boil. Reduce heat to low and simmer 20 minutes, stirring occasionally.

4. Divide evenly among six airtight containers. Store in the refrigerator until ready to eat.

PER SERVING Calories: 416 | Fat: 29 g | Protein: 25 g | Sodium: 656 mg | Fiber: 4.5 g | Carbohydrates: 13 g | Sugar: 2.5 g

Broccoli Cheddar Soup

If you want to change this soup up a little bit, you can swap out the Cheddar and use another kind of cheese or you can use a combination of your favorites. You can keep this soup in the refrigerator up to 1 week.

INGREDIENTS | SERVES 6

1 tablespoon olive oil
3 cloves garlic, minced
¼ cup minced yellow onion
4 cups broccoli florets, finely chopped
3½ cups no-sugar-added chicken broth
1 cup coconut cream
3 cups shredded Cheddar cheese

1. Heat olive oil in a large stockpot over medium heat. Add garlic and onions and cook until translucent, about 4 minutes.

2. Add broccoli, chicken broth, and coconut cream. Bring mixture to a boil and then reduce heat to low and allow to simmer 20 minutes or until broccoli is tender.

3. Keeping the heat on low, add cheese ½ cup at a time, stirring as you add and waiting until cheese is fully melted and incorporated into soup to add more.

4. Divide evenly among six airtight containers. Store in the refrigerator until ready to eat.

PER SERVING Calories: 427 | Fat: 35 g | Protein: 21 g | Sodium: 492 mg | Fiber: 3 g | Carbohydrates: 10 g | Sugar: 3 g

Chicken Minestrone Soup

This is a good soup to work into your meal plan at the end of the week or when you're trying to use up any leftover vegetables. You can add any low-carb vegetables that you have on hand to eliminate waste and free up room in your refrigerator. It will last up to 1 week in the refrigerator.

INGREDIENTS | SERVES 6

2 tablespoons olive oil

½ medium yellow onion, peeled and diced

2 cloves garlic, minced

3 stalks celery, chopped

1 medium zucchini, diced

1 cup green beans, chopped in ½" pieces

1 tablespoon Italian seasoning

4 cups no-sugar-added chicken broth

1 (14-ounce) can crushed tomatoes

2 (12.5-ounce) cans shredded chicken

½ teaspoon salt

¼ teaspoon freshly ground black pepper

1. Heat olive oil in large stockpot over medium heat. Add onion, garlic, and celery and cook until tender, about 5 minutes. Add zucchini and green beans and cook 2 more minutes.

2. Add remaining ingredients and bring to a boil. Reduce heat to low and allow to simmer 1 hour.

3. Divide evenly among six airtight containers. Store in the refrigerator until ready to eat.

PER SERVING   Calories: 312 | Fat: 15 g | Protein: 34 g | Sodium: 909 mg | Fiber: 3 g | Carbohydrates: 10 g | Sugar: 4 g

Cold Green Soup

Because this soup is made for you to enjoy cold, it's a great option when you're not going to have access to a stove to reheat your food. It will keep in the refrigerator for 1 week.

INGREDIENTS | SERVES 6

3 cups baby spinach

1 large avocado, pitted and peeled

1 large cucumber, peeled

¾ cup chopped red bell pepper

½ cup vegetable broth

2 cloves garlic

1 tablespoon coconut aminos

1 tablespoon lemon juice

2 tablespoons chopped scallions

¼ teaspoon salt

⅛ teaspoon freshly ground black pepper

⅛ teaspoon crushed red pepper flakes

1. Combine all ingredients in a blender. Blend until smooth. Serve cold.

2. Divide evenly among six airtight containers. Store in the refrigerator until ready to eat.

PER SERVING   Calories: 115 | Fat: 6 g | Protein: 3.5 g | Sodium: 295 mg | Fiber: 3 g | Carbohydrates: 13 g | Sugar: 3 g

Spicy Pumpkin Soup

Be sure to use canned pumpkin purée or freshly puréed pumpkin for this recipe. Avoid canned pumpkin pie filling, which has sugar added to it and a significantly higher carbohydrate count than pure pumpkin. This soup will last 1 week in the refrigerator.

INGREDIENTS | SERVES 6

2 tablespoons olive oil

1 small white onion, peeled and diced

2 cloves garlic, minced

2 tablespoons minced chipotle in adobo sauce

1 teaspoon ground cumin

1 teaspoon ground coriander

⅛ teaspoon ground cloves

⅛ teaspoon pumpkin pie spice

¾ teaspoon salt

¼ teaspoon freshly ground black pepper

2 cups puréed pumpkin

4 cups no-sugar-added chicken broth

½ cup full-fat coconut milk

1 teaspoon smoked paprika (optional)

1. Heat olive oil in a medium stockpot over medium heat. Add onions and garlic and cook until translucent, about 4 minutes. Add chipotle and spices and cook another 3 minutes.

2. Add pumpkin purée and chicken broth to pot, stir, and allow to simmer 5 minutes.

3. Use an immersion blender to purée ingredients. Add coconut milk, purée again, and allow to simmer 5 more minutes.

4. Divide evenly among six airtight containers. Store in the refrigerator until ready to eat. Sprinkle each portion with paprika before serving if desired.

PER SERVING Calories: 138 | Fat: 10 g | Protein: 5 g | Sodium: 346 mg | Fiber: 3 g | Carbohydrates: 10 g | Sugar: 3 g

Vitamin A–Packed Pumpkin

Pumpkin gets a lot of attention in the fall months, but the nutrient-rich squash should be a part of your diet all year. Pumpkin is one of the richest sources of vitamin A, which keeps your vision strong, helps your nerves function normally, and protects the health of your skin. A half cup of puréed pumpkin provides three times the amount of vitamin A that you need for the entire day.

Cheeseburger Soup

This recipe makes a creamy, cheesy soup, but if you want a soup that's more broth-like, you can omit the coconut cream and sprinkle some cheese on top after you heat it up but right before you eat. You can keep this soup in the refrigerator up to 1 week.

INGREDIENTS | SERVES 6

2 tablespoons olive oil

3 cloves garlic, minced

1 large yellow onion, peeled and diced

1 pound 80/20 ground beef

3 medium yellow squash, seeded and diced

2 (15-ounce) cans diced tomatoes

3 cups beef broth

1 teaspoon salt

1 teaspoon freshly ground black pepper

1 tablespoon Italian seasoning

1 teaspoon garlic powder

1 teaspoon onion powder

⅓ cup coconut cream

1¼ cups shredded Cheddar cheese

1. Heat olive oil in a large stockpot over medium heat. Add garlic and onion and cook until translucent, about 4 minutes. Add ground beef and cook until no longer pink, about 7 minutes.

2. Add squash, tomatoes, broth, and seasonings and stir to combine. Bring to a boil and then turn heat to low and allow to simmer 1 hour. Add coconut cream and cheese and allow to simmer 30 more minutes.

3. Divide evenly among six airtight containers. Store in the refrigerator until ready to eat.

PER SERVING   Calories: 372 | Fat: 25 g | Protein: 25 g | Sodium: 1,023 mg | Fiber: 4 g | Carbohydrates: 12 g | Sugar: 7 g

Cauliflower Chowder

If you want to save some time, use frozen cauliflower for this recipe. You won't have to do any chopping, and the softer texture is perfect for a chowder. This chowder can keep up to 1 week in the refrigerator.

INGREDIENTS | SERVES 6

3 slices no-sugar-added bacon, chopped

2 tablespoons ghee

2 cloves garlic, minced

1 medium yellow onion, peeled and diced

3 stalks celery, diced

1 large head cauliflower, chopped into small pieces

¼ cup almond flour

4 cups no-sugar-added chicken broth

1 cup unsweetened almond milk

1 teaspoon salt

½ teaspoon freshly ground black pepper

2 tablespoons minced fresh parsley

Flat Leaf versus Curly Parsley

There are two kinds of parsley available: flat leaf and curly. Both may be used in any recipe, but flat leaf parsley typically has a more robust flavor and minces finer than curly parsley, which has a tougher texture. If you want the parsley to blend into the dish better, choose flat leaf.

1. Heat a large stockpot over medium heat and add bacon. Cook until crispy, about 7 minutes. Remove from pot and place on plate lined with paper towel.

2. Melt ghee in stockpot and add garlic, onions, and celery. Cook until tender, about 4 minutes.

3. Add cauliflower and cook until it just starts to soften, about 4 minutes. Whisk in flour until slightly browned, about 2 minutes, and continue whisking as you add chicken broth and almond milk. Keep whisking until mixture starts to thicken, about 5 minutes.

4. Bring to a boil and then reduce heat and simmer 15 minutes or until cauliflower is tender. Stir in remaining ingredients.

5. Divide evenly among six airtight containers. Store in the refrigerator until ready to eat.

PER SERVING Calories: 200 | Fat: 12 g | Protein: 9 g | Sodium: 605 mg | Fiber: 3 g | Carbohydrates: 16 g | Sugar: 5 g

(Almost) Zuppa Toscana Soup

This soup is a low-carb copycat of the famous Zuppa Toscana soup at the Olive Garden. It has all the delicious flavor with none of the ingredients that you don't want. It will keep for 1 week in the refrigerator.

INGREDIENTS | SERVES 6

½ pound no-sugar-added bacon, diced

1 pound ground no-sugar-added pork sausage

2 tablespoons olive oil

3 cloves garlic, minced

1 medium yellow onion, peeled and diced

6 cups no-sugar-added chicken broth

4 cups finely chopped cauliflower

1½ cups full-fat coconut milk

4 cups kale, chopped into bite-sized pieces

1. Heat a medium skillet over medium heat and cook bacon until crispy, about 6 minutes. Scoop bacon out of skillet with slotted spoon and transfer to a plate lined with a paper towel.

2. Add sausage to skillet with bacon grease and cook until no longer pink, about 8 minutes. Set aside.

3. Heat olive oil in a large stockpot over medium heat. Add garlic and onions and cook until translucent, about 4 minutes.

4. Add bacon and sausage. Then add chicken broth and cauliflower and stir until combined. Cook 20 minutes or until cauliflower is tender.

5. Stir in coconut milk and kale and simmer another 10 minutes.

6. Divide evenly among six airtight containers. Store in the refrigerator until ready to eat.

PER SERVING Calories: 659 | Fat: 56 g | Protein: 29 g | Sodium: 420 mg | Fiber: 2 g | Carbohydrates: 12 g | Sugar: 3 g

Chicken and Mushroom Soup

If you want to freeze this soup, skip adding the coconut milk for now. You can freeze in individual portions and then stir ⅓ cup coconut milk into each portion right before eating. It will keep up to 1 week in the refrigerator.

INGREDIENTS | SERVES 6

½ cup ghee

2 stalks celery, chopped

1 small white onion, peeled and minced

2 cloves garlic, minced

½ pound boneless, skinless chicken breasts, cut into 1" cubes

1 pound sliced baby bella mushrooms

3 cups no-sugar-added chicken broth

1 teaspoon salt

½ teaspoon freshly ground black pepper

½ teaspoon dried rosemary

½ teaspoon dried thyme

2 cups full-fat coconut milk

1. Melt ghee in a large stockpot over medium heat. Add celery, onion, and garlic and cook until softened, about 4 minutes. Add chicken and cook until no longer pink, about 7 minutes.

2. Add mushrooms and cook until softened, about 2 minutes. Pour in broth, salt, pepper, rosemary, and thyme. Bring to a boil and then reduce heat to low and simmer 25 minutes.

3. Stir in coconut milk.

4. Divide evenly among six airtight containers. Store in the refrigerator until ready to eat.

PER SERVING Calories: 388 | Fat: 35 g | Protein: 15 g | Sodium: 472 mg | Fiber: 1.5 g | Carbohydrates: 8 g | Sugar: 2 g

Thymol in Thyme

Thyme is one of the most versatile herbs on the planet—it's used for everything from cooking to incense to essential oils to mouthwash. The powerful herb contains an oil called thymol, which has extremely powerful antiseptic and antibacterial properties. One study found that thyme's antibacterial properties are so strong that the oil extracted from it can kill methicillin-resistant Staphylococcus aureus, more commonly referred to as MRSA.

Beef Stew

Beef chuck is commonly used in stews and slow cooker recipes that call for beef, but you can also use bottom round roast, rump round, top round, and pot roast with equally delicious results. Whatever you choose, this stew will last up to 1 week in the refrigerator.

INGREDIENTS | SERVES 6

3 tablespoons olive oil, divided

1 cup whole mushrooms, quartered

1 medium yellow onion, peeled and chopped

3 cloves garlic, minced

2 medium carrots, peeled and cut in ½" rounds

4 stalks celery, chopped

2 pounds beef chuck, cut into cubes

2 tablespoons tomato paste

1½ teaspoons salt

1 teaspoon freshly ground black pepper

½ teaspoon dried thyme

4 cups beef broth

1 teaspoon coconut aminos

1. Heat 1 tablespoon olive oil in a large stockpot over medium heat. Add mushrooms and toss to coat in oil. Let cook 2 minutes without stirring. Stir and then cook 2 minutes more. Remove mushrooms from pot and set aside.

2. Add another tablespoon olive oil to pot and heat over medium heat. Add onions, garlic, carrots, and celery and cook until tender, about 5 minutes. Remove from pot and set aside with mushrooms.

3. Heat remaining oil in pot over medium heat and brown the beef in batches, cooking about 3 minutes on each side. Once all beef is browned, add it to the pot along with tomato paste, salt, pepper, and thyme, making sure all beef gets coated. Cook 2 minutes and then add cooked vegetables and stir.

4. Slowly pour beef broth into pot while gently scraping the browned pieces from the bottom of the pot. Add coconut aminos, stir, and allow to simmer 1 hour.

5. Divide evenly among six airtight containers. Store in the refrigerator until ready to eat.

PER SERVING Calories: 334 | Fat: 17 g | Protein: 34 g | Sodium: 1,074 mg | Fiber: 2 g | Carbohydrates: 7 g | Sugar: 3 g

Cauliflower Cheddar Soup

The jicama in this soup adds some texture after the soup is blended. If you can't find any jicama, you can use turnips in its place. This soup will keep in the refrigerator up to 1 week.

INGREDIENTS | SERVES 6

2 tablespoons ghee

1 cup diced white onion

3 stalks celery, chopped

3 cloves garlic, minced

1 cup diced jicama

6 cups no-sugar-added chicken broth

4 cups chopped cauliflower florets

1 teaspoon dried thyme

1 teaspoon salt

¼ teaspoon freshly ground black pepper

1 cup shredded Cheddar cheese

1 teaspoon coconut aminos

Get to Know Jicama

Jicama, also known as the Mexican yam bean or Mexican turnip, is widely underused and underappreciated. Like potatoes, jicamas are root vegetables, but they are significantly lower in carbohydrates. One cup of jicama contains only 11 carbohydrates, 6 of which come from fiber, while 1 cup of white potatoes contains 26 grams of carbohydrates, only 1.5 of which come from fiber. Jicamas have a similar texture to white potatoes, although they're a little crispier, and they make a great low-carb substitution in soups.

1. Heat ghee in a large stockpot over medium heat. Add onion, celery, and garlic and cook until celery is softened, about 5 minutes.

2. Add all remaining ingredients except cheese and coconut aminos. Bring to a boil over high heat and then reduce heat to low and allow to simmer 20 minutes or until cauliflower is tender.

3. Blend the soup with an immersion blender until completely smooth. Stir in cheese and coconut aminos.

4. Divide evenly among six airtight containers. Store in the refrigerator until ready to eat.

PER SERVING   Calories: 210 | Fat: 13 g | Protein: 12 g | Sodium: 674 mg | Fiber: 3.5 g | Carbohydrates: 12 g | Sugar: 3 g

Mulligatawny Soup

If you use a medium Granny Smith apple in this recipe, it will only add about 2.5 grams of carbohydrates to each serving, but if you're concerned about meeting your carbohydrate goals, you can leave it out. This soup will keep up to 1 week in the refrigerator.

INGREDIENTS | SERVES 6

2 tablespoons ghee

1 medium yellow onion, peeled and chopped

1 cup chopped celery

1 medium carrot, peeled and diced

1 small green pepper, seeded and minced

1 medium Granny Smith apple, peeled and diced

1 tablespoon freshly grated ginger

3 tablespoons coconut flour

1 teaspoon arrowroot powder

1 teaspoon lemon juice

2 tablespoons curry powder

8 cups no-sugar-added chicken broth

1 pound boneless, skinless chicken breasts, cooked and shredded

1 teaspoon salt

¼ teaspoon freshly ground black pepper

¾ cup full-fat coconut milk

1. Heat ghee in a large stockpot over medium heat. Add onions, celery, carrots, green pepper, apple, and ginger. Sauté until softened, about 5 minutes.

2. Stir in coconut flour, arrowroot powder, lemon juice, and curry powder and cook another 3 minutes.

3. Add all remaining ingredients except coconut milk and bring to a boil. Reduce heat to low and allow to simmer 1 hour.

4. Stir in coconut milk and allow to simmer 5 more minutes. Remove from heat and allow to cool.

5. Divide evenly among six airtight containers. Store in the refrigerator until ready to eat.

PER SERVING Calories: 269 | Fat: 14 g | Protein: 25 g | Sodium: 546 mg | Fiber: 4.5 g | Carbohydrates: 13 g | Sugar: 2 g

What Is Mulligatawny Soup?

Mulligatawny soup is an English soup with Indian roots. One thing that mulligatawny soups usually have in common is their traditional curry flavor, but there are many variations on the classic. Some are made with chicken, while others are made with lamb. Some have legumes, rice, and carrots, while others are designed to be low-carb.

Creamy Vegetable Soup

If you prefer a broth-based soup, you can leave out the coconut milk and still end up with a delicious soup that holds up well in the refrigerator for up to 1 week. If you want the best of both worlds, add a little coconut milk to the soup after you heat it up right before eating.

INGREDIENTS | SERVES 6

2 tablespoons ghee

1 small yellow onion, peeled and diced

2 cloves garlic, minced

½ cup diced celery

2 quarts chicken stock

2 cups chopped cauliflower florets

2 cups chopped broccoli florets

½ teaspoon dried oregano

½ teaspoon dried rosemary

1 teaspoon salt

1 teaspoon freshly ground black pepper

½ cup full-fat coconut milk

Fill Up Your Freezer

Frozen cauliflower and broccoli are ideal for this recipe because they're already chopped, and you can keep them in your freezer at all times so they're always on hand.

1. Heat ghee in a large stockpot over medium heat. Add onions and garlic and cook until they start to soften, about 3 minutes. Add celery and cook 3 more minutes.

2. Add chicken stock, cauliflower, broccoli, herbs, salt, and pepper and turn heat to high. Bring to a boil, reduce heat to low, and allow to simmer 20 minutes.

3. When vegetables are done simmering, use an immersion blender to purée or transfer soup to a high-speed blender in batches.

4. After soup is puréed, stir in coconut milk.

5. Divide soup evenly into six airtight containers and store in the refrigerator until ready to eat.

PER SERVING Calories: 218 | Fat: 12 g | Protein: 10 g | Sodium: 877 mg | Fiber: 2 g | Carbohydrates: 17 g | Sugar: 6 g

Creamy Brussels Sprouts Soup

Once you try this soup, it will become your favorite new way to eat Brussels sprouts. It freezes really well, so don't be afraid to make a double batch and save some for later. You can store it in the freezer up to 3 months and in the refrigerator up to 1 week.

INGREDIENTS | SERVES 6

4 tablespoons ghee

3 cloves garlic, minced

3 (10-ounce) packages frozen Brussels sprouts, thawed and chopped

3 slices no-sugar-added bacon, diced

3 cups no-sugar-added chicken broth

2½ cups full-fat coconut milk

½ teaspoon oregano

¼ teaspoon paprika

½ teaspoon salt

¼ teaspoon freshly ground black pepper

½ cup shredded white Cheddar cheese

1. Heat ghee in a large stockpot over medium heat. Add garlic and cook 1 minute. Add Brussels sprouts and bacon and cook until bacon is crisp and Brussels sprouts are caramelized, about 10 minutes.

2. Stir in remaining ingredients except cheese and bring to a boil. Reduce heat to low and simmer 20 minutes. Stir in cheese.

3. Divide evenly among six airtight containers. Store in the refrigerator until ready to eat.

PER SERVING Calories: 442 | Fat: 39 g | Protein: 14 g | Sodium: 420 mg | Fiber: 5 g | Carbohydrates: 16 g | Sugar: 0 g

Cream of Zucchini Soup

The sour cream in this recipe makes the soup a little creamier, but if you want to make this recipe dairy-free, you can leave it out and still have a delicious result. This soup will last 1 week in the refrigerator.

INGREDIENTS | SERVES 6

1 medium yellow onion, peeled and chopped

3 cloves garlic, roughly chopped

4 medium zucchini, roughly chopped

4 cups no-sugar-added chicken broth

½ teaspoon salt

¼ teaspoon freshly ground black pepper

3 tablespoons sour cream

1. Combine all ingredients except sour cream in a large stockpot and bring to a boil over medium-high heat. Reduce heat to low, cover, and allow to simmer 20 minutes or until zucchini is tender.

2. Remove from heat and purée with an immersion blender. Stir in sour cream.

3. Divide evenly among six airtight containers. Store in the refrigerator until ready to eat.

PER SERVING Calories: 69 | Fat: 2.5 g | Protein: 5 g | Sodium: 256 mg | Fiber: 2 g | Carbohydrates: 8 g | Sugar: 4 g

Gazpacho

Classic gazpacho uses fresh vine-ripened tomatoes, but this version, which is made with canned tomatoes, actually holds up better in the refrigerator, so it's perfect as part of your low-carb meal prep menu. This dish will last up to 6 days in the refrigerator.

INGREDIENTS | SERVES 6

2 (14.5-ounce) cans petite diced tomatoes, divided

½ cup water

2 tablespoons olive oil

½ cup peeled and diced English cucumber

1 small red bell pepper, seeded and finely diced

¼ cup minced green onion

2 cloves garlic, minced

1 small jalapeño, seeded and diced

1 teaspoon salt

½ teaspoon freshly ground black pepper

2 tablespoons lime juice

1. Combine ½ cup tomatoes, water, and olive oil in a blender or food processor. Process until smooth.

2. Transfer to a medium bowl and add remaining ingredients. Stir to mix well.

3. Divide evenly among six airtight containers. Store in the refrigerator until ready to eat.

PER SERVING Calories: 72 | Fat: 5 g | Protein: 2 g | Sodium: 535 mg | Fiber: 2 g | Carbohydrates: 7 g | Sugar: 4 g

Slow Cooker Meals

Cauliflower Leek Soup

Choose leeks that have a lot of white and pale green, which are the only edible parts. You'll only be using the white portion for this recipe, but you can reserve the pale green portion for a soup or stock. Be sure to discard the dark green portion—it's fibrous and inedible. You can store this soup in the refrigerator up to 1 week.

INGREDIENTS | SERVES 6

4 large leeks, white part only, chopped

1 (16-ounce) bag frozen cauliflower

3 stalks celery, diced

1½ teaspoons salt

¾ teaspoon freshly ground black pepper

3 cloves garlic, minced

4 cups no-sugar-added chicken broth

1 cup unsweetened coconut milk

½ cup shredded Parmesan cheese

1. Combine all ingredients except Parmesan cheese in a slow cooker. Cover and cook on low 7 hours or high 3 hours.

2. Add Parmesan cheese and use an immersion blender to blend until smooth.

3. Divide into six equal portions and store each portion in a separate airtight container in the refrigerator until ready to eat.

PER SERVING   Calories: 135 | Fat: 10 g | Protein: 7 g | Sodium: 710 mg | Fiber: 2 g | Carbohydrates: 8 g | Sugar: 2 g

Chicken Enchilada Soup

You can use a taco seasoning packet for this recipe, but make sure that it doesn't contain anything other than spices. Some taco seasonings have corn starch, wheat, and sugar, which can affect the carbohydrate count and make this soup less nutritious. Store soup in the refrigerator up to 1 week.

INGREDIENTS | SERVES 6

1½ pounds boneless, skinless chicken breasts

1 medium yellow onion, peeled and diced

1 medium green bell pepper, seeded and diced

½ medium jalapeño, seeded and diced

2 cloves garlic, minced

1 (15-ounce) can diced fire-roasted tomatoes

2 cups no-sugar-added chicken broth

1 tablespoon chili powder

1 tablespoon cumin

1 teaspoon paprika

1 teaspoon dried oregano

½ teaspoon crushed red pepper flakes

1. Line the bottom of a slow cooker with chicken breasts. Add remaining ingredients and gently stir until combined, making sure chicken breasts stay in place.

2. Cover and cook on low 8 hours. Shred chicken with a fork and stir to combine. Divide into six equal portions and store each portion in a separate airtight container in the refrigerator until ready to eat.

PER SERVING   Calories: 171 | Fat: 3.5 g | Protein: 27 g | Sodium: 156 mg | Fiber: 2 g | Carbohydrates: 6 g | Sugar: 3 g

Mexican Pot Roast

This Mexican Pot Roast pairs extremely well with Cauliflower "Rice" (Chapter 13) and a basic green salad. Whip up a batch of Enchilada Sauce (Chapter 9), pour it on top before storing your portions for the week, and you're ready to go. Store in the refrigerator up to 1 week.

INGREDIENTS | SERVES 6

2 teaspoons granulated garlic

1 teaspoon granulated onion

1 teaspoon ground cumin

½ teaspoon paprika

¼ teaspoon oregano

1 teaspoon salt

1 teaspoon freshly ground black pepper

3½ pounds chuck roast

3 tablespoons ghee

3 tablespoons tomato paste

1 tablespoon coconut aminos

2 cups no-sugar-added salsa

1 cup beef broth

Easy Fresh Salsa

If you can't find jarred salsa without added sugar, you can quickly whip up your own fresh salsa by combining 3 cups chopped tomatoes, ½ cup diced red onion, ½ cup diced green pepper, ¼ cup minced cilantro, 1 small diced jalapeño pepper, 2 tablespoons lime juice, 1 minced garlic clove, ½ teaspoon salt, ½ teaspoon black pepper, and ½ teaspoon cumin in food processor and pulsing to mix well.

1. Combine granulated garlic, granulated onion, cumin, paprika, oregano, salt, and pepper in a small bowl. Rub spice mixture all over chuck roast, covering as much as possible.

2. Heat ghee in a medium skillet over medium-high heat. Brown roast on all sides (cook about 2 minutes per side) and then transfer roast to a slow cooker.

3. Mix tomato paste and coconut aminos and pour over roast. Add salsa and beef broth and cover.

4. Cook on high 1 hour and then reduce heat to low and continue cooking 6 hours or until roast is tender.

5. When roast is tender, transfer to a cutting board and shred using two forks. Add shredded meat back to slow cooker and stir in juices.

6. Divide evenly among six airtight containers and store in the refrigerator until you're ready to eat.

PER SERVING Calories: 505 | Fat: 25 g | Protein: 58 g | Sodium: 1,093 mg | Fiber: 2.5 g | Carbohydrates: 10 g | Sugar: 5 g

Beef and Broccoli

Chuck roast is a great slow-cooking meat because it's a tough cut that contains a lot of collagen. When slow cooked, the collagen breaks down into gelatin, which tenderizes the meat and adds lots of flavor. This completed dish will keep in the refrigerator up to 1 week.

INGREDIENTS | SERVES 6

1 cup beef broth

½ cup coconut aminos

2 tablespoons sesame oil

2 cloves garlic, minced

1 teaspoon freshly grated ginger

1 teaspoon salt

½ teaspoon freshly ground black pepper

½ teaspoon arrowroot powder

1½ pounds boneless beef chuck roast

2 cups chopped broccoli florets

1. Add beef broth, coconut aminos, sesame oil, garlic, ginger, salt, pepper, and arrowroot powder to a slow cooker. Whisk to combine.

2. Put chuck roast on top and cover. Cook on low 4–6 hours or until beef is tender and comes apart easily with a fork.

3. Add broccoli florets to slow cooker, cover, and cook on low another 10 minutes or until broccoli is tender.

4. Remove roast from slow cooker, shred with two forks, and return to slow cooker. Toss to coat beef and broccoli with sauce.

5. Divide evenly among six airtight containers and store in the refrigerator until you're ready to eat.

PER SERVING Calories: 237 | Fat: 12 g | Protein: 25 g | Sodium: 1,075 mg | Fiber: 0 g | Carbohydrates: 3 g | Sugar: 1 g

Easy Chicken Thighs

If you find yourself in a jam with frozen chicken thighs, you can make this recipe in your pressure cooker instead. All you have to do is add all the ingredients to your pot, cook on high pressure for 20 minutes, and release pressure manually. These thighs will keep up to 1 week in the refrigerator.

INGREDIENTS | SERVES 6

¼ cup coconut aminos

1 cup no-sugar-added chicken broth

½ teaspoon granulated garlic

½ teaspoon ground ginger

½ teaspoon salt

½ teaspoon freshly ground black pepper

1½ pounds boneless, skinless chicken thighs

1. Combine coconut aminos, chicken broth, garlic, and ginger in a slow cooker.

2. Rub salt and pepper on chicken thighs and put in slow cooker with broth mixture.

3. Cover and cook on high 5 hours or until chicken is tender and cooked through.

4. Divide evenly among six airtight containers and store in the refrigerator until you're ready to eat.

PER SERVING   Calories: 152 | Fat: 5 g | Protein: 23 g | Sodium: 501 mg | Fiber: 0 g | Carbohydrates: 2 g | Sugar: 0 g

Chicken Marinara Casserole

This casserole tastes even better on days two and three than it does on day one. It's a good recipe to make in advance because the flavors meld together as it sits in the refrigerator over the week and the acid from the tomatoes does its magic. Store in the refrigerator up to 1 week.

INGREDIENTS | SERVES 6

2 (8-ounce) cans no-sugar-added tomato sauce

1 (4-ounce) can tomato paste

2 cloves garlic, minced

2 teaspoons dried basil

2 teaspoons dried oregano

½ teaspoon salt

¼ teaspoon freshly ground black pepper

1½ pounds boneless, skinless chicken breasts, cubed

¾ cup shredded mozzarella cheese

1. Add tomato sauce, tomato paste, garlic, basil, oregano, salt, and pepper to a slow cooker and stir to combine. Add cubed chicken and toss to coat.

2. Cover and cook on low 4 hours or until chicken is tender and cooked through.

3. Divide into six equal portions and sprinkle ⅛ cup shredded cheese on each portion.

4. Store in an airtight container in the refrigerator until ready to eat.

PER SERVING   Calories: 215 | Fat: 6 g | Protein: 30 g | Sodium: 845 mg | Fiber: 2 g | Carbohydrates: 8 g | Sugar: 5 g

Coconut Chicken Curry

If you prefer to make this recipe nut-free, you can swap out the peanut butter and use sunflower seed butter, which is similar in both taste and texture. If you're okay with nuts but want to avoid peanuts, you can use almond butter instead. This curry will last up to 1 week in the refrigerator.

INGREDIENTS | SERVES 6

1 (13.5-ounce) can full-fat coconut milk

1 teaspoon curry powder

⅛ teaspoon ground turmeric

¼ teaspoon crushed red pepper flakes

¼ teaspoon ground ginger

¼ teaspoon salt

¼ teaspoon freshly ground black pepper

2 tablespoons no-sugar-added creamy peanut butter

2 tablespoons coconut aminos

½ cup chopped yellow onion

½ cup sliced yellow bell pepper

⅓ cup chopped cilantro

6 (4-ounce) boneless, skinless chicken breasts

1. Combine coconut milk, curry powder, turmeric, red pepper flakes, ginger, salt, pepper, peanut butter, and coconut aminos in slow cooker and stir to combine.

2. Add onion, bell pepper, and cilantro and stir.

3. Place chicken breasts in curry sauce and cook on low 6 hours or until chicken is cooked and tender. Shred chicken with a fork and mix to combine with sauce.

4. Divide evenly among six airtight containers and store in the refrigerator until you're ready to eat.

PER SERVING Calories: 156 | Fat: 14 g | Protein: 3 g | Sodium: 272 mg | Fiber: 1 g | Carbohydrates: 5 g | Sugar: 2 g

Cleansing with Cilantro

Cilantro is a natural blood cleanser. It helps remove toxins from the blood by supporting the body's natural detoxification systems (the kidneys, liver, and digestive system). The herb also acts as a diuretic, helping you shed excess water weight and lose the bloat.

Pulled Pork Chili

The fire-roasted tomatoes in this recipe give it a little extra kick and some added flavor, but if you only have regular diced tomatoes on hand, you can double up on those instead. This chili can last up to 1 week in the refrigerator.

INGREDIENTS | SERVES 6

2 tablespoons paprika

2 tablespoons chili powder

1 tablespoon garlic powder

1 teaspoon cayenne pepper

1 teaspoon crushed red pepper flakes

½ teaspoon oregano

1 teaspoon salt

2 pounds pork shoulder

2 cloves garlic, minced

½ cup Frank's RedHot

1 large white onion, peeled and chopped

1 medium red bell pepper, seeded and diced

1 medium yellow bell pepper, seeded and diced

1 medium green bell pepper, seeded and diced

1 (15-ounce) can diced fire-roasted tomatoes

1 (15-ounce) can petite diced tomatoes

1 (15-ounce) can no-sugar-added tomato sauce

1. Combine paprika, chili powder, garlic powder, cayenne pepper, red pepper flakes, oregano, and salt in a small bowl. Rub spice mixture over pork shoulder, covering as much as possible.

2. Put pork shoulder in slow cooker. Add remaining ingredients and cover. Cook 8–10 hours on low or until pork is cooked through and tender.

3. Shred pork with a fork and stir to combine.

4. Divide evenly among six airtight containers and store in the refrigerator until you're ready to eat.

PER SERVING Calories: 221 | Fat: 9 g | Protein: 25 g | Sodium: 463 mg | Fiber: 4 g | Carbohydrates: 11 g | Sugar: 6 g

Pork Roast

If you have extra time during your meal prep, you can rub the pork shoulder with the dry rub, wrap it in plastic wrap, and refrigerate it a few hours or overnight. This allows the flavors to penetrate the meat a little more. This recipe will keep in the refrigerator up to 1 week.

INGREDIENTS | SERVES 12

1 teaspoon chili powder

1 teaspoon cumin

½ teaspoon onion powder

½ teaspoon garlic powder

½ teaspoon paprika

½ teaspoon salt

½ teaspoon freshly ground black pepper

3 pounds pork shoulder

¼ cup coconut aminos

1. Mix spices together in a small bowl. Rub spice blend over pork shoulder and completely cover.

2. Add pork shoulder to slow cooker and pour coconut aminos over it.

3. Cook on low 6 hours or until pork shreds easily with a fork.

4. Divide half the meat evenly among six airtight containers and store in the refrigerator until you're ready to eat. Store the rest in a freezer-safe container and freeze up to 3 months.

PER SERVING   Calories: 172 | Fat: 8 g | Protein: 22 g | Sodium: 333 mg | Fiber: 0 g | Carbohydrates: 1 g | Sugar: 0 g

Jerk Chicken

Jerk chicken is known for its kick, but if you prefer something a bit less spicy, just reduce or omit the cayenne pepper from this recipe. This chicken will last up to 1 week in the refrigerator.

INGREDIENTS | SERVES 6

3 teaspoons salt

2 teaspoons freshly ground black pepper

3 teaspoons paprika

2 teaspoons garlic powder

2 teaspoons onion powder

1 teaspoon thyme

1 teaspoon cayenne pepper

1½ pounds chicken thighs, bone in and skin on

1. Combine spices in a large bowl. Add chicken thighs and toss to coat completely.

2. Layer chicken in slow cooker and cook on low 5–6 hours or until chicken is tender and no longer pink.

3. Remove from heat and transfer 4 ounces of chicken to each of six airtight containers. Store in the refrigerator until ready to eat.

PER SERVING   Calories: 148 | Fat: 5 g | Protein: 22 g | Sodium: 1,271 mg | Fiber: 1 g | Carbohydrates: 3 g | Sugar: 0 g

Shrimp Scampi

Cutting something crosswise means instead of cutting it from the root end to the bud end (which would be lengthwise), you cut it down its circumference or right in the middle at the largest point. This scampi will keep in the refrigerator up to 3 days.

INGREDIENTS | SERVES 6

2 cups no-sugar-added chicken broth

1 teaspoon arrowroot powder

1 small yellow onion, peeled and diced

2 cloves garlic, minced

2 teaspoons lemon garlic seasoning

2 tablespoons ghee

1 (3-pound) spaghetti squash, cut in half crosswise and seeded

36 jumbo shrimp (about 1½ pounds), peeled and deveined

Use What You've Got!

Instead of throwing away the seeds you remove from the spaghetti squash, you can roast them and eat them as a snack or add them to your Mason jar salads. To roast, clean squash guts from seeds and pat dry. Place seeds in a small bowl and coat with olive oil and salt. The proper ratio is about 1 tablespoon olive oil and ½ teaspoon salt per cup of seeds. Spread seeds out on a parchment paper–lined baking sheet and bake at 275°F about 15–20 minutes or until seeds start to pop.

1. Combine all ingredients except spaghetti squash and shrimp in the slow cooker and stir. Put spaghetti squash, cut side down, into slow cooker. Cook on high 2 hours or until spaghetti squash is tender.

2. Add shrimp to the slow cooker and cook covered 20 more minutes.

3. Once shrimp is cooked, use oven mitts to remove spaghetti squash from slow cooker. Allow to cool and then use a fork to remove squash from skin.

4. Toss cooked shrimp with spaghetti squash and sauce. Divide scampi evenly into six airtight containers and store in the refrigerator.

PER SERVING Calories: 163 | Fat: 5 g | Protein: 10 g | Sodium: 271 mg | Fiber: 3.5 g | Carbohydrates: 18 g | Sugar: 5 g

Sausage and Peppers

You can use sweet or hot sausage for this recipe; just make sure it doesn't have any sugar added to it. It may be slightly difficult to find at your local grocery store, but your butcher may be able to make you some by special request, if necessary. You can keep this up to 1 week in the refrigerator.

INGREDIENTS | SERVES 6

5 cloves garlic, minced

2 teaspoons salt

½ teaspoon basil

½ teaspoon oregano

¼ teaspoon thyme

¼ teaspoon crushed red pepper flakes

1 (28-ounce) can crushed tomatoes

¼ cup vegetable broth

2 large yellow onions, peeled and thinly sliced

2 medium green bell peppers, seeded and thinly sliced

1 medium red bell pepper, seeded and thinly sliced

1 medium orange bell pepper, seeded and thinly sliced

1½ pounds no-sugar-added Italian sausage links

1. Add garlic, spices, tomatoes, and vegetable broth to slow cooker and stir to mix well. Add onions and peppers and toss to make sure they're evenly coated.

2. Bury sausage links underneath onion and pepper mixture and cover. Cook on low 5–6 hours or until sausage is cooked through and onions and peppers are tender.

3. Allow to cool and evenly distribute sausage and peppers among six airtight containers. Store in the refrigerator until you're ready to eat.

PER SERVING   Calories: 534 | Fat: 45 g | Protein: 29 g | Sodium: 341 mg | Fiber: 0 g | Carbohydrates: 3 g | Sugar: 1 g

Beef Stroganoff

This beef stroganoff pairs extremely well with the Cauliflower Mash (Chapter 10). When planning your meals for the week, you may want to make both of these at the same time. You can store them together in the same container in the refrigerator up to 1 week for an easy, complete meal.

INGREDIENTS | SERVES 6

2 teaspoons salt

1 teaspoon freshly ground black pepper

1 teaspoon garlic powder

1 teaspoon paprika

1 teaspoon chili powder

1 teaspoon onion powder

2 pounds chuck roast, cut into 1" cubes

2 tablespoons olive oil

1 small yellow onion, peeled and finely diced

8 ounces sliced baby bella mushrooms

⅓ cup coconut cream

2 teaspoons coconut aminos

1 teaspoon red wine vinegar

1. Combine spices in a medium mixing bowl. Add cubed meat and toss to coat.

2. Spread olive oil in slow cooker, add onions and mushrooms, and put beef on top. Cover and cook on low 4–5 hours or until beef is tender.

3. Once beef is cooked, add remaining ingredients and cook on high an additional hour.

4. Allow to cool slightly and then divide beef stroganoff evenly into six airtight containers. Store in the refrigerator until ready to eat.

PER SERVING   Calories: 321 | Fat: 18 g | Protein: 33 g | Sodium: 922 mg | Fiber: 1 g | Carbohydrates: 5 g | Sugar: 2 g

Corned Beef and Cabbage

Most corned beef comes with a prepared spice packet that you can use to season the beef. If the ingredients fall into your healthy, low-carb plan, you can use the included spice packet instead of the spices listed in this recipe. If it contains any sugar or artificial ingredients, stick with this recipe. This will keep up to 1 week in the refrigerator.

INGREDIENTS | SERVES 6

1½ pounds corned beef

1 large white onion, peeled and roughly chopped

4 cups water

2 tablespoons apple cider vinegar

1 teaspoon minced garlic

1 teaspoon whole black peppercorns

½ teaspoon mustard seeds

¼ teaspoon crushed red pepper flakes

2 bay leaves

1 small head cabbage, roughly chopped

1. Place corned beef in the bottom of a slow cooker and surround with onions.

2. Pour water and vinegar over beef and onions and mix in spices. Cover and cook on low 4 hours. Add cabbage and cook another 60–90 minutes or until cabbage is tender.

3. Remove corned beef from slow cooker and cut into slices. Divide slices evenly among six airtight containers. Add cabbage and a spoonful of liquid to containers. Store in the refrigerator until you're ready to eat.

PER SERVING   Calories: 330 | Fat: 16 g | Protein: 32 g | Sodium: 1,037 mg | Fiber: 4 g | Carbohydrates: 11 g | Sugar: 6 g

Chicken Curry

This recipe is so easy it's almost criminal. If you're new to meal prep, this recipe will save a lot of hassle as you get the hang of spending a couple hours in the kitchen. This dish keeps up to 1 week in the refrigerator.

INGREDIENTS | SERVES 6

1 cup full-fat coconut milk

2 tablespoons red curry paste

¼ teaspoon turmeric

1½ pounds boneless, skinless chicken breasts

What's in Red Curry Paste?

Red curry paste is a combination of red chili, garlic, lemongrass, Thai ginger, salt, shallots, coriander, and lime leaf. You can also use green curry paste, which contains green chili as a main ingredient, in the place of red for a different flavor profile.

1. Add coconut milk, curry paste, and turmeric to slow cooker and stir with a fork until curry is fully incorporated. Add chicken and toss to coat.

2. Cook on low 4–5 hours or until chicken comes apart easily with a fork. Shred chicken, stir, and allow to cook 20 more minutes.

3. Remove chicken from slow cooker with a slotted spoon and transfer 4 ounces to each of six airtight containers. Store in the refrigerator until you're ready to eat.

PER SERVING Calories: 216 | Fat: 11 g | Protein: 26 g | Sodium: 56 mg | Fiber: 1 g | Carbohydrates: 2 g | Sugar: 0 g

Garlic Shrimp

This isn't your typical set-it-and-forget-it slow cooker recipe. There are short periods of downtime, but you'll need to be around to do the steps. While the shrimp cooks in the slow cooker, you can prepare your other recipes and come back to this one to finish it off. Store this dish in the refrigerator for 3 days.

INGREDIENTS | SERVES 6

¾ cup olive oil

2 tablespoons ghee

5 cloves garlic, thinly sliced

½ teaspoon paprika

¼ teaspoon garlic powder

¼ teaspoon onion powder

1 teaspoon salt

¼ teaspoon freshly ground black pepper

⅛ teaspoon cayenne pepper

36 jumbo shrimp (about 1½ pounds), peeled and deveined

1. Set slow cooker to high and add olive oil, ghee, garlic, and spices. Stir until ghee is melted and all ingredients are combined. Cover and allow to cook 30 minutes.

2. Add shrimp to slow cooker and stir to evenly coat. Cook 25 minutes covered, stirring halfway through.

3. When shrimp are done cooking, transfer six shrimp to each of six airtight containers and pour sauce evenly on top of shrimp. Store in the refrigerator.

PER SERVING Calories: 310 | Fat: 31 g | Protein: 9 g | Sodium: 438 mg | Fiber: 0 g | Carbohydrates: 1 g | Sugar: 0 g

Balsamic Chicken

While it's not necessary to spend a fortune on imported, aged balsamic vinegar, make sure to get one that's truly balsamic vinegar. Check the ingredient list. Ideally, you want to see grapes and maybe some vinegar. You don't want to see sugar, artificial flavors, and/or coloring agents. This chicken will keep up to 1 week in the refrigerator.

INGREDIENTS | SERVES 6

1 teaspoon garlic powder

1 teaspoon onion powder

½ teaspoon salt

½ teaspoon freshly ground black pepper

1 teaspoon dried minced onion

1½ pounds boneless, skinless chicken thighs

3 cloves garlic, minced

2 tablespoons olive oil

⅓ cup balsamic vinegar

1. In a small bowl, combine garlic powder, onion powder, salt, pepper, and minced onion. Rub dry spice mixture on each chicken thigh, coating as much as possible.

2. Place chicken thighs in slow cooker.

3. In a separate small bowl, combine minced garlic, olive oil, and balsamic vinegar and stir to mix well. Pour over chicken in slow cooker.

4. Cover and cook on low 6 hours.

5. Allow chicken to cool and then divide evenly among six airtight containers. Store in the refrigerator until you're ready to eat.

PER SERVING   Calories: 190 | Fat: 9 g | Protein: 22 g | Sodium: 303 mg | Fiber: 0 g | Carbohydrates: 3 g | Sugar: 2 g

Italian Meatloaf

Many store-bought ketchups are full of sugar or, even worse, high-fructose corn syrup. This recipe calls for homemade Ketchup (Chapter 9). If you're able to find a store-bought ketchup that doesn't contain any added sugar or artificial sweeteners, you can use that as well. This meatloaf will keep in the refrigerator for 1 week.

INGREDIENTS | SERVES 6

1½ pounds ground beef
2 large eggs
1 cup shredded zucchini, strained
¼ cup grated Parmesan cheese
¼ cup parsley, chopped
3 cloves garlic, minced
2 tablespoons coconut aminos
1 tablespoon dried minced onion
½ teaspoon salt
½ teaspoon freshly ground black pepper
¾ cup Ketchup (Chapter 9), divided

1. Combine all ingredients except ½ cup ketchup in a medium bowl and use your hands to mix thoroughly.

2. Line the bottom of the slow cooker with two pieces of aluminum foil, making sure foil comes up the sides of the slow cooker so you can lift meatloaf out when it's done.

3. Place mixture on top of prepared foil and shape it into a meatloaf. Cover and cook on low 6 hours.

4. Once meatloaf is cooked, spread remaining ketchup on top, cover, and cook 10 more minutes.

5. Remove meatloaf from slow cooker by lifting aluminum foil. Allow to rest. Once meatloaf is cool, cut into six equal portions and place each portion in an airtight container. Refrigerate until ready to eat.

PER SERVING Calories: 285 | Fat: 14 g | Protein: 26 g | Sodium: 822 mg | Fiber: 0 g | Carbohydrates: 12 g | Sugar: 8 g

Zucchini in a Meatloaf?

Most meatloaf recipes call for bread crumbs. Even healthier versions that replace the bread crumbs with oats can be too high in carbohydrates. The zucchini in this recipe gives the meatloaf the added moisture it needs and helps hold it together so that it doesn't fall apart. Make sure you squeeze out the excess water, though. Zucchini is 95 percent water, so if you don't remove some of it, the meatloaf could come out watery.

Sausage-Stuffed Peppers

This recipe can be made with any color bell pepper without changing the carbohydrate count significantly. Feel free to use your favorite or a mixture of all colors. These peppers will keep up to 1 week in the refrigerator.

INGREDIENTS | SERVES 6

1 pound ground hot no-sugar-added Italian sausage

1½ cups riced cauliflower

1 (8-ounce) can tomato paste

1 small yellow onion, peeled and diced

2 cloves garlic, minced

1½ tablespoons Italian seasoning

6 medium red bell peppers, tops cut off and seeds scooped out

¼ cup water

1. Combine all ingredients except peppers and water in a medium bowl and mix thoroughly. You might have to use your hands to make sure everything is fully incorporated.

2. Stuff each pepper with equal amounts of sausage mixture. Pour water into the bottom of the slow cooker, place stuffed peppers in water, and loosely put tops back in place.

3. Cook on low 6 hours or until sausage is fully cooked.

4. Remove from slow cooker and transfer each stuffed pepper to an airtight container. Refrigerate until you're ready to eat.

PER SERVING Calories: 294 | Fat: 19 g | Protein: 14 g | Sodium: 860 mg | Fiber: 4 g | Carbohydrates: 18 g | Sugar: 11 g

Taco Meat

Basic taco meat is a low-carb meal prep staple. It's super simple, it tastes great with lots of sides, and it freezes well, so you can whip up a big batch and save some for later. This prepared meat will last in the refrigerator up to 1 week.

INGREDIENTS | SERVES 6

1 tablespoon chili powder

1½ teaspoons ground cumin

½ teaspoon paprika

1 teaspoon salt

1 teaspoon freshly ground black pepper

¼ teaspoon oregano

¼ teaspoon crushed red pepper flakes

¼ teaspoon granulated onion

¼ teaspoon granulated garlic

1½ pounds ground beef

2 tablespoons tomato paste

1. Combine spices in a small bowl and stir to mix well.

2. Add ground beef, spices, and tomato paste to the slow cooker. Use a wooden spoon to mix and break up the beef.

3. Cook on low 4 hours. Stir to break up meat, then remove from slow cooker with a slotted spoon.

4. Transfer 4 ounces of prepared taco meat to each of six airtight containers. Store in the refrigerator until you're ready to eat.

PER SERVING Calories: 209 | Fat: 11 g | Protein: 23 g | Sodium: 544 mg | Fiber: 1 g | Carbohydrates: 2.5 g | Sugar: 0 g

Pressure Cooker Meals

Easy Shredded Chicken

This recipe is perfect for meal prep because it's basic, and you can use it for any of the recipes that call for shredded chicken. Cook up a batch and use it to make a bunch of Mason jar salads or just have it on hand when you need a quick protein fix. This chicken will last 1 week in the refrigerator.

INGREDIENTS | SERVES 8

1 teaspoon salt
½ teaspoon freshly ground black pepper
2 pounds boneless, skinless chicken breasts
¼ cup no-sugar-added chicken broth

Manual Release versus Natural Release

These pressure cooker recipes are designed for an electric pressure cooker. Each recipe will specify either manual release or natural release. With manual pressure release, you turn the steam valve after cooking, and the pressure will come rushing out of the top of the pressure cooker in the form of steam. With natural release, you leave the pressure cooker alone and let the pressure release slowly from the valve on its own. Either way, there's no need to worry, because the pressure cooker has a safety feature that won't allow you to open it until the pressure has been adequately released.

1. Sprinkle salt and pepper on chicken breasts.

2. Pour chicken broth into pressure cooker pot and put trivet in place. Pile chicken on trivet and close pressure cooker lid.

3. Cook on high pressure 20 minutes. After 20 minutes, release pressure manually.

4. Remove chicken from pressure cooker and use two forks to shred.

5. Use chicken immediately as part of your meal prep recipe or store in an airtight container in the refrigerator to use later.

PER SERVING Calories: 134 | Fat: 3 g | Protein: 25 g | Sodium: 341 mg | Fiber: 0 g | Carbohydrates: 0 g | Sugar: 0 g

Steamed Artichokes

Don't let artichokes scare you. They may be a little strange looking, but they're simple to whip up in a pressure cooker, and the hearts make a fabulous low-carb addition to your Mason jar salads. These artichokes will keep in the refrigerator up to 1 week.

INGREDIENTS | SERVES 4

4 teaspoons olive oil

1 teaspoon lemon juice

2 teaspoons minced garlic

¼ teaspoon salt

4 medium artichokes, tops cut off crosswise

½ cup water

1. In a small bowl, combine olive oil, lemon juice, garlic, and salt. Use a pastry or basting brush to spread equal amounts of olive oil mixture on top of each artichoke.

2. Pour water in the bottom of pressure cooker pot and put trivet in place. Place artichokes cut side up on trivet.

3. Close lid and cook 8 minutes. When artichokes are done cooking, release pressure manually.

4. Divide into six equal portions and store each portion in a separate airtight container in the refrigerator until ready to eat.

PER SERVING Calories: 68 | Fat: 3 g | Protein: 3 g | Sodium: 177 mg | Fiber: 4 g | Carbohydrates: 9 g | Sugar: 1 g

"Hard-Boiled" Eggs

This recipe calls for 12 eggs, but depending on the size of your pressure cooker, you may be able to fit up to 24 at once. You can increase the number of eggs without having to change anything else in this recipe. These eggs will last 1 week in the refrigerator.

INGREDIENTS | SERVES 6

1 cup water

12 large eggs

Peel Now or Later?

It's usually easiest to peel hard-boiled eggs right after cooling them before storage, but if you prefer to leave the shell on until you're ready to eat, that's okay too. The cooked eggs will last in your refrigerator for up to 1 week whether they are peeled or not.

1. Pour water into pressure cooker pot. Put trivet in place.

2. Carefully place eggs on trivet and close lid.

3. Cook on high pressure 4 minutes. As soon as eggs are done cooking, release pressure manually.

4. Transfer eggs from pressure cooker into a large bowl of ice water and let cool 5 minutes.

5. Use in your meal prep recipe or put eggs in an airtight container and store in the refrigerator until ready to eat.

PER SERVING Calories: 143 | Fat: 9 g | Protein: 12.5 g | Sodium: 142 mg | Fiber: 0 g | Carbohydrates: 0 g | Sugar: 0 g

Basic Spaghetti Squash

Spaghetti squash is a low-carb diet staple, and with this recipe, you can have some cooked and ready to go in under 30 minutes. Whip some up just to have on hand or use this squash for the other recipes that call for cooked squash. This squash will keep up to 1 week in the refrigerator.

INGREDIENTS | SERVES 6

1 cup water

1 medium spaghetti squash (about 3 pounds), cut in half crosswise, with guts and seeds removed

Squash Too Big?

If you can't fit your entire spaghetti squash in your pressure cooker, you can cook one half at a time. Just cut the squash crosswise and then cut each half crosswise again, so you have four pieces. Cook two pieces at a time.

1. Pour water into the bottom of a pressure cooker and then put trivet in place. Place spaghetti squash cut side down on trivet.

2. Put pressure cooker lid in place and cook on high pressure 8 minutes. After 8 minutes, release pressure manually.

3. Remove spaghetti squash with oven mitts. (It will be very hot!) Allow to cool slightly and then remove squash strands from skin with a fork.

4. Use cooked spaghetti squash in your recipe or transfer to an airtight container and store in the refrigerator until ready to eat.

PER SERVING   Calories: 39 | Fat: 0 g | Protein: 1 g | Sodium: 4 mg | Fiber: 2 g | Carbohydrates: 10 g | Sugar: 2 g

Cauliflower "Rice"

The most common way to prepare cauliflower rice is to shred the cauliflower florets with a food processor. This pressure cooker version allows you to quickly make cauliflower rice, and unlike the food processor method, this way gives you rice that's already cooked! This rice will last up to 1 week in the refrigerator.

INGREDIENTS | SERVES 6

1 cup no-sugar-added chicken broth

1 large head cauliflower, cut into large florets

2 tablespoons ghee

1 teaspoon salt

½ teaspoon freshly ground black pepper

Make It Your Own

This recipe is for basic cauliflower rice, but it's easily adaptable to your tastes. You can make it your own by adding different combinations of spices, like garlic salt or taco seasoning.

1. Pour chicken broth into pot insert. Put trivet in place.

2. Add cauliflower to pot and close lid. Cook on high pressure 1 minute.

3. Immediately release pressure manually and remove cauliflower from pot, lifting up by the trivet.

4. Pour out excess chicken broth and return insert to pressure cooker. Turn to Sauté function and add ghee. Return cooked cauliflower to pot and break apart using a potato masher. The goal is to get small, rice-like pieces, not to mash the cauliflower, so do this part carefully. Sprinkle with salt and pepper and stir gently.

5. Remove cauliflower from pressure cooker and transfer evenly to six airtight containers. Store in refrigerator until ready to eat.

PER SERVING   Calories: 68 | Fat: 4 g | Protein: 3 g | Sodium: 429 mg | Fiber: 2 g | Carbohydrates: 5 g | Sugar: 2 g

Beef Barbacoa

Chipotle peppers are smoke-dried jalapeños, which means they have all the spice as well as a little smoke. When chopping peppers, make sure to use gloves to avoid skin irritation. You can keep this beef in the refrigerator up to 1 week.

INGREDIENTS | SERVES 6

1 medium yellow onion, peeled and sliced

5 cloves garlic, smashed

2 (4-ounce) cans green chilies

2 medium dried chipotle peppers, stems removed and coarsely chopped

½ teaspoon salt

½ teaspoon freshly ground black pepper

¼ teaspoon ground cloves

1 teaspoon cumin

1 teaspoon oregano

Juice from 2 medium limes, about 3–4 tablespoons

2 tablespoons apple cider vinegar

½ cup beef broth

2 pounds beef brisket

1. Add all ingredients except beef to pressure cooker pot and stir to combine. Place beef in liquid and close lid.

2. Cook on high pressure 60 minutes. When beef is done cooking, allow pressure to release naturally.

3. Remove lid, use two forks to shred beef, and stir. Turn pressure cooker back to Sauté and allow the juices to reduce, stirring frequently.

4. After juices have reduced, about 30 minutes, transfer shredded beef in equal portions to six airtight containers and store in the refrigerator until ready to eat.

PER SERVING   Calories: 260 | Fat: 10 g | Protein: 33 g | Sodium: 353 mg | Fiber: 1 g | Carbohydrates: 6 g | Sugar: 2 g

Spicy Sausage and Escarole Soup

This recipe has a kick, especially if you use the sausage spice blend listed in this recipe. If you want to dial it down a notch, reduce or omit the crushed red pepper and cayenne pepper. This soup will keep in the refrigerator for up to 1 week.

INGREDIENTS | SERVES 6

1 tablespoon olive oil

1 large yellow onion, peeled and diced

2 tablespoons minced garlic

1 pound no-sugar-added pork sausage

4½ cups no-sugar-added chicken broth

¼ cup chopped fresh parsley

1 large bunch escarole, coarsely chopped

1 teaspoon salt

1 teaspoon freshly ground black pepper

½ teaspoon crushed red pepper flakes

Pork Sausage Blend

Sometimes it can be difficult to find pork sausage without any added sugar or undesirable ingredients. To make your own, combine 1 teaspoon salt, ½ teaspoon dried parsley, ¼ teaspoon ground sage, ¼ teaspoon ground black pepper, ¼ teaspoon dried thyme, ¼ teaspoon crushed red pepper flakes, ⅛ teaspoon ground cayenne pepper, and ¼ teaspoon ground coriander in a small bowl. Mix into ground pork thoroughly before cooking.

1. Use Sauté function to heat olive oil. Add onions and garlic and cook until translucent, about 4 minutes. Add pork and cook until no longer pink, about 7 minutes.

2. Add remaining ingredients and stir to combine. Cover and make sure vent is closed.

3. Set Soup function to 20 minutes and start cook time.

4. When timer goes off, allow pressure to release naturally. Remove pressure cooker lid and allow to cool. Once cooled, divide evenly and store each portion in an airtight container in the refrigerator until ready to eat.

PER SERVING Calories: 325 | Fat: 24 g | Protein: 20 g | Sodium: 512 mg | Fiber: 0.5 g | Carbohydrates: 6 g | Sugar: 1 g

Whole Chicken with Gravy

This recipe makes lots of extra gravy. After you prepare this dish for the week, you can freeze the rest of the gravy and save it for another time. In addition to giving this chicken an extra kick, it goes really well on top of the Cauliflower Mash (Chapter 10). Store in the refrigerator up to 1 week.

INGREDIENTS | SERVES 6

1½ teaspoons salt

1 teaspoon freshly ground black pepper

1 teaspoon granulated garlic

½ teaspoon paprika

3 tablespoons avocado oil, divided

1 (4-pound) whole chicken

2 large yellow onions, peeled and roughly chopped

5 cloves garlic, peeled and mashed

½ cup no-sugar-added chicken broth

1 tablespoon arrowroot powder

1 tablespoon water

1. In a small bowl, combine salt, pepper, granulated garlic, paprika, and 2 tablespoons avocado oil. Stir to mix well.

2. Rub oil mixture all over chicken, covering as much as you can, inside and out.

3. Turn pressure cooker on to Sauté setting. Once it gets hot, place chicken, breast side down, in pot. Allow chicken to cook about 4 minutes or until skin starts to get a little brown and crisp. Flip chicken over and do the same on the other side. Remove chicken from pot and set aside.

4. Heat remaining tablespoon avocado oil and add onion and garlic. Cook until they start to soften, about 4 minutes. Add chicken broth and stir.

5. Place trivet in pot and put seared chicken, breast side up, on trivet. Close lid and cook on high pressure 20 minutes.

6. When chicken is done cooking, release pressure manually. Remove chicken from pot and allow to rest.

7. While chicken is resting, use an immersion blender to blend contents of pot. If you don't have an immersion blender, you can pour contents into a blender and make the gravy that way.

8. Combine arrowroot powder and water and mix well. Stir into gravy to thicken.

9. Carve chicken and divide evenly among six airtight containers. Pour 2 tablespoons gravy on top of chicken and store in the refrigerator until ready to eat.

PER SERVING Calories: 220 | Fat: 10 g | Protein: 24 g | Sodium: 647 mg | Fiber: 1 g | Carbohydrates: 6 g | Sugar: 2 g

Buttery Lemon Chicken

One of the perks of using a pressure cooker is that you can use frozen meat without thawing. If you're using frozen chicken for this recipe, all you have to do is increase cooking time to 15 minutes. This chicken will last up to 1 week in the refrigerator.

INGREDIENTS | SERVES 6

1 teaspoon salt

½ teaspoon freshly ground black pepper

¾ teaspoon paprika

½ teaspoon granulated onion

1½ pounds boneless, skinless chicken breasts

2 tablespoons ghee

3 cloves garlic, minced

1 medium yellow onion, peeled and diced

½ cup no-sugar-added chicken broth

¼ cup lemon juice

3 teaspoons arrowroot powder

3 teaspoons water

1. Combine salt, pepper, paprika, and granulated onion in a small bowl. Season both sides of each chicken breast.

2. Turn on Sauté function of pressure cooker and add ghee to pot. Once ghee is heated, add garlic and onion and sauté until softened, about 4 minutes. Add chicken breast and sear, about 3 minutes on each side.

3. Pour chicken broth and lemon juice in pot and close lid. Cook 7 minutes on high pressure. Let pressure release naturally.

4. Remove chicken from pot and divide evenly among six airtight containers.

5. Mix arrowroot powder and water and then stir into contents of pressure cooker to thicken sauce. Pour sauce evenly over chicken.

6. Store chicken in refrigerator until ready to eat.

PER SERVING Calories: 185 | Fat: 7 g | Protein: 25 g | Sodium: 445 mg | Fiber: 0 g | Carbohydrates: 3 g | Sugar: 1 g

Chicken Curry and Turnips

This recipe requires some advance preparation, so make sure to plan for that when using it as part of your meal prep. You can prepare the marinade the night before you're ready to cook and let the chicken sit in it overnight if it makes things easier. This cooked chicken dish will last up to 1 week in the refrigerator.

INGREDIENTS | SERVES 6

1 teaspoon garlic powder

1 teaspoon onion powder

2 teaspoons curry powder

1 teaspoon salt

1 tablespoon olive oil

1½ pounds boneless, skinless chicken breasts

2 tablespoons ghee

1 cup full-fat coconut milk

1½ teaspoons curry powder

3 cups peeled and diced turnips

1 teaspoon granulated erythritol

1 teaspoon arrowroot powder

1 teaspoon water

The Low-Carb Root Vegetable

Turnips and potatoes are both root vegetables, but turnips have significantly fewer carbohydrates. A half cup of diced white potatoes contains 13 grams of carbohydrates, whereas a half cup diced turnips contains only 4.2 grams, but because of their similar taste, you won't even notice the difference!

1. Combine garlic powder, onion powder, curry powder, salt, and olive oil in a medium bowl. Stir to mix well. Add chicken breasts to bowl, making sure chicken is coated and submerged as much as possible. Cover and allow chicken to sit in marinade in the refrigerator 1 hour.

2. Turn pressure cooker on to Sauté function and add ghee to pot. Allow to heat and then add marinated chicken breast, searing about 3 minutes on each side.

3. Add coconut milk, curry powder, turnips, and erythritol to pot and close lid. Cook on high pressure 25 minutes. When done cooking, release pressure manually.

4. Open pot and remove chicken with a slotted spoon. Combine arrowroot powder and water in a small bowl and pour into curry mixture in the pot. Stir until thickened.

5. Divide chicken evenly among six airtight containers and pour sauce and turnips over each breast. Store in the refrigerator until ready to eat.

PER SERVING   Calories: 290 | Fat: 17 g | Protein: 26 g | Sodium: 487 mg | Fiber: 2 g | Carbohydrates: 7 g | Sugar: 2.5 g

Beef Shawarma

Beef shawarma is a Lebanese dish that involves cooking meat for hours on a spit, similar to the way gyros are prepared. Although this dish isn't technically shawarma since it's prepared in a pressure cooker, the flavors are reminiscent of the traditional dish. You can store this in the refrigerator up to 1 week.

INGREDIENTS | SERVES 6

1½ pounds ground beef

1 large yellow onion, peeled and thinly sliced

1 small head cabbage, roughly chopped

1 cup diced red bell pepper

1 teaspoon salt

1½ teaspoons dried oregano

¾ teaspoon ground cumin

¾ teaspoon ground coriander

¼ teaspoon cardamom

¼ teaspoon cayenne pepper

¾ teaspoon ground cinnamon

¼ teaspoon ground allspice

1. Turn pressure cooker on to Sauté function. Add ground beef to pot and cook until just browned, making sure to adequately break up meat. You don't have to cook it completely.

2. Add remaining ingredients and cook on high 3 minutes. Allow the pressure to release naturally.

3. Divide beef evenly among six airtight containers and store in the refrigerator until ready to eat.

PER SERVING Calories: 252 | Fat: 11 g | Protein: 24 g | Sodium: 490 mg | Fiber: 4 g | Carbohydrates: 12 g | Sugar: 7 g

The Perfect Pairing

This Beef Shawarma goes exceptionally well with Tzatziki Sauce (Chapter 9), or you can make a simple dressing for it by combining 2 teaspoons of tahini, ½ cup of lemon juice, 3 cloves crushed garlic, and ½ teaspoon salt.

Chicken and Kale Soup

If you have prepared Easy Shredded Chicken (see recipe in this chapter), you can use that in place of this cubed chicken breast. If you do, you can reduce cooking time to 5 minutes since the chicken is already cooked. This soup will keep up to 1 week in the refrigerator.

INGREDIENTS | SERVES 6

2 tablespoons ghee

2 cloves garlic, minced

1 medium yellow onion, peeled and diced

4 stalks celery, diced

1½ pounds boneless, skinless chicken breasts, cubed

6 cups no-sugar-added chicken broth

1 cup peeled and cubed turnips

2 cups chopped kale

1 teaspoon fish sauce

1 teaspoon salt

1 teaspoon freshly ground black pepper

½ teaspoon dried thyme

¼ teaspoon dried rosemary

¼ teaspoon dried sage

1. Turn pressure cooker on to Sauté function and add ghee to pot. When ghee is hot, add garlic, onion, and celery and sauté until softened, about 4 minutes. Add cubed chicken and stir to brown each side. (You don't have to cook it completely.)

2. Add remaining ingredients, close lid, turn pressure cooker to Soup function, and set the time for 20 minutes.

3. When soup is done cooking, allow pressure to release naturally.

4. Allow soup to cool slightly. Divide evenly among six airtight containers and store in the refrigerator until ready to eat.

PER SERVING Calories: 235 | Fat: 8 g | Protein: 31 g | Sodium: 585 mg | Fiber: 2 g | Carbohydrates: 8 g | Sugar: 2.5 g

Pork Roast with Gravy

If your pork roast is frozen, there is no need to thaw! That's the beauty of a pressure cooker. Follow this recipe exactly as is but increase the cooking time to 90 minutes. This cooked roast will last up to 1 week in the refrigerator.

INGREDIENTS | SERVES 6

2 tablespoons ghee

1 medium yellow onion, peeled and roughly chopped

3 cloves garlic, roughly chopped

2 stalks celery, diced

4 cups chopped cauliflower florets

2 cups beef broth

1 teaspoon salt

½ teaspoon freshly ground black pepper

2 pounds pork shoulder

Alternate Option

Instead of using cauliflower and turning the vegetables into gravy, you can use 4 cups of cubed turnips in this recipe. When everything is done cooking, remove meat, scoop turnips out of the liquid with a slotted spoon, and store until you're ready to eat.

1. Turn pressure cooker on to Sauté function and add ghee. When ghee is hot, add onion, garlic, and celery and sauté until softened, about 4 minutes.

2. Add cauliflower to pot, pour in beef broth, stir in salt and pepper, and set pork shoulder on top.

3. Close lid and cook on high pressure 60 minutes. Release pressure manually.

4. Remove pork from pot and set aside to rest. While pork is resting, use an immersion blender to blend cauliflower and beef broth mixture into gravy. If you don't have an immersion blender, transfer contents to a blender or food processor and process until smooth.

5. Shred pork using two forks. Transfer pork evenly to six airtight containers and top meat with gravy. Store in the refrigerator until ready to eat.

PER SERVING Calories: 299 | Fat: 15 g | Protein: 31 g | Sodium: 840 mg | Fiber: 1.5 g | Carbohydrates: 5 g | Sugar: 2 g

Italian Wedding Soup

This is another recipe with an easy, quick preparation that freezes very well. If your pressure cooker has the extra space, consider doubling up when you make this and freezing some for your meals down the road. This soup will keep up to 1 week in the refrigerator.

INGREDIENTS | SERVES 6

1 pound ground no-sugar-added Italian sausage

1 tablespoon ghee

1 large yellow onion, peeled and chopped

2 cloves garlic, minced

4 cups no-sugar-added chicken broth

½ teaspoon salt

½ teaspoon freshly ground black pepper

¼ teaspoon onion powder

¼ teaspoon dried basil

3 cups chopped spinach

1. Shape sausage into twenty-four equal-sized mini meatballs. Set aside.

2. Turn pressure cooker on to Sauté function and add ghee. When ghee is heated, add onion and garlic and sauté until softened, about 4 minutes. Add meatballs and allow to brown. Turn and allow to brown some more, about 2 minutes.

3. Add remaining ingredients except spinach, stir, and close lid. Choose the Manual setting and set time to 5 minutes. After soup finishes cooking, allow pressure to release naturally. Open lid and stir in spinach while soup is hot.

4. Allow soup to cool and then divide evenly into six airtight containers. Store in the refrigerator until ready to eat.

PER SERVING Calories: 274 | Fat: 21 g | Protein: 15 g | Sodium: 807 mg | Fiber: 1 g | Carbohydrates: 6 g | Sugar: 2 g

Chicken and Summer Squash Soup

Bok choy, also called Chinese cabbage, is a leafy vegetable with round leaves on large white stalks. When choosing bok choy, look for dark green leaves that are crisp and have no visible wilting or brown spots. This soup will keep up to 1 week in the refrigerator.

INGREDIENTS | SERVES 6

1 tablespoon ghee

1 small shallot, minced

2 cloves garlic, minced

1½ pounds boneless, skinless chicken breasts, cubed

2 quarts no-sugar-added chicken broth

1 large zucchini, diced

1 large yellow squash, diced

1 large vine-ripened tomato, diced

1 cup chopped asparagus

2 cups chopped bok choy leaves

Juice from 1 medium lemon, about 2 tablespoons

½ teaspoon dried rosemary

1 teaspoon dried thyme

1 teaspoon salt

½ teaspoon freshly ground black pepper

1. Turn pressure cooker on to Sauté setting and add ghee to pot. When ghee is hot, add shallots and garlic and sauté until softened, about 3 minutes.

2. Add chicken and cook 3–4 minutes, browning on each side. Add 1 cup chicken broth and stir to scrape browned bits from bottom of pot.

3. Pour in remaining chicken broth and all other ingredients.

4. Close lid, turn pressure cooker to Soup setting, and set time for 12 minutes. When soup is done cooking, allow pressure to release naturally.

5. Allow soup to cool and then divide among six airtight containers and store in the refrigerator until ready to eat.

PER SERVING   Calories: 232 | Fat: 7 g | Protein: 33 g | Sodium: 557 mg | Fiber: 2 g | Carbohydrates: 9 g | Sugar: 4 g

Benefits of Bok Choy

Bok choy belongs to the cruciferous family of vegetables, which also includes broccoli, kale, cauliflower, Brussels sprouts, and cabbage. One cup of bok choy contains only 9 calories and 1.5 grams of carbohydrates but provides 62 percent of your daily vitamin A and 52 percent of your vitamin C.

Cabbage Soup

To prepare cabbage, strip the outer leaves, wash the cabbage, then slice into quarters. Remove the hard core on each quarter, then roughly chop and measure. This soup will keep up to 1 week in the refrigerator.

INGREDIENTS | SERVES 6

1 tablespoon olive oil

½ medium yellow onion, peeled and diced

2 cloves garlic, minced

1½ pounds ground beef

½ teaspoon ground cumin

1 teaspoon salt

½ teaspoon freshly ground black pepper

1 large head green cabbage, roughly chopped

1 (4-ounce) can green chilies

1 small vine-ripened tomato, diced

2 teaspoons tomato paste

6 cups beef broth

1. Turn pressure cooker on to Sauté function and add olive oil. When olive oil is hot, add onions and garlic and cook until softened, about 4 minutes. Add ground beef, cumin, salt, and pepper and cook until beef is no longer pink, about 7 minutes.

2. Add remaining ingredients, stir to combine, and close lid.

3. Choose Soup setting and cook 20 minutes. Allow pressure to release naturally.

4. After pot is depressurized, allow soup to cool and divide evenly into six airtight containers. Store in the refrigerator until ready to eat.

PER SERVING Calories: 289 | Fat: 14 g | Protein: 27 g | Sodium: 901 mg | Fiber: 4.5 g | Carbohydrates: 13 g | Sugar: 7 g

Bacon Chili

Tomato-based meals like this chili are extremely stable in the refrigerator and the freezer. If you have a large pressure cooker, you can double this recipe and freeze half of it to save for later. After cooking, transfer half the cooked chili to a freezer-safe container and store up to 3 months or keep in the refrigerator for 1 week.

INGREDIENTS | SERVES 6

6 slices no-sugar-added bacon, roughly chopped

2 cloves garlic, minced

1 large yellow onion, peeled and diced

2 medium red bell peppers, seeded and diced

1 pound ground beef

½ pound ground turkey

1 tablespoon chili powder

1 tablespoon paprika

1 tablespoon garlic powder

1½ teaspoons cumin

1½ teaspoons onion powder

½ teaspoon salt

½ teaspoon freshly ground black pepper

1 (14-ounce) can fire-roasted tomatoes

1 (15-ounce) can no-sugar-added tomato sauce

1. Turn pressure cooker on to Sauté function and add bacon to pot. Sauté until bacon is crispy. Remove bacon and discard all but 1 tablespoon of bacon fat.

2. Add garlic, onions, and peppers to bacon fat and sauté until softened, about 5 minutes.

3. Return bacon to pot, add all remaining ingredients, stir to combine, and close pressure cooker lid.

4. Choose Chili setting and set time to 30 minutes. When chili is done cooking, allow pressure to release naturally.

5. Allow chili to cool and then divide into six equal portions and place each portion in an airtight container. Store in the refrigerator until ready to eat.

PER SERVING   Calories: 370 | Fat: 22 g | Protein: 28 g | Sodium: 707 mg | Fiber: 4.5 g | Carbohydrates: 14 g | Sugar: 7 g

Chicken Tikka Masala

This is a traditional Indian dish that combines chunks of chicken with a creamy, spicy tomato sauce. This version is made quickly and easily in a pressure cooker, and the flavors get even better the longer it sits in your refrigerator! It can stay in your refrigerator up to 1 week.

INGREDIENTS | SERVES 6

2 tablespoons olive oil

1 large yellow onion, peeled and diced

2 cloves garlic, minced

1 tablespoon minced fresh ginger

2 teaspoons paprika

2 teaspoons cumin

1 teaspoon garam masala

1 teaspoon ground turmeric

1 teaspoon ground coriander

½ teaspoon ground cayenne pepper

½ teaspoon salt

1 (8-ounce) can no-sugar-added tomato sauce

½ cup no-sugar-added chicken broth

1½ pounds boneless, skinless chicken breasts

½ cup full-fat coconut milk

Juice from 1 medium lemon, about 2 tablespoons

1. Turn pressure cooker on to Sauté function and add olive oil to pot. When olive oil is hot, add onion, garlic, and ginger and sauté until softened, about 4 minutes. Add spices to onion mixture and stir to mix well.

2. Add tomato sauce, chicken broth, and chicken and stir. Close lid, select Manual function, and cook on high pressure 8 minutes. Release pressure manually, open pressure cooker, and remove chicken.

3. Shred chicken with two forks and then return to pot. Stir in coconut milk and lemon juice.

4. Allow to cool and then divide evenly among six airtight containers. Store in the refrigerator until ready to eat.

PER SERVING   Calories: 243 | Fat: 12 g | Protein: 27 g | Sodium: 432 mg | Fiber: 1.5 g | Carbohydrates: 7 g | Sugar: 2.5 g

Make Your Own Garam Masala

You can purchase garam masala already made for you, but it's easy to make your own with spices you probably already have on hand. Combine 2 tablespoons ground cumin, 3 teaspoons ground coriander, 3 teaspoons ground cardamom, 3 teaspoons black pepper, 2 teaspoons ground cinnamon, 1 teaspoon ground cloves, and 1 teaspoon ground nutmeg in a small bowl and stir to mix well. Store in an airtight container in a cool, dry place.

Chicken Poblano Soup

If you want a spicier soup, use red poblano peppers. If you want a milder soup, use green poblano peppers. Or use a combination of both for a soup that's somewhere in the middle. You can keep this soup in the refrigerator up to 1 week.

INGREDIENTS | SERVES 6

2 tablespoons ghee

1 small yellow onion, peeled and diced

3 medium poblano peppers, roughly chopped

4 cloves garlic, mashed

2 cups chopped cauliflower

1 small vine-ripened tomato, diced

1 (6-ounce) can green chilies

1½ pounds boneless, skinless chicken thighs

¼ cup chopped cilantro

1 teaspoon ground coriander

1 teaspoon ground cumin

¼ teaspoon dried oregano

1 teaspoon salt

3 cups no-sugar-added chicken broth

Kick the Flavor Up a Notch

If you have a little extra time and you want to kick the flavor of this soup up a notch, you can roast the poblano peppers before chopping and adding them to your pressure cooker. To roast, set oven to 425°F, rub peppers in a light layer of olive oil, place on a baking sheet, and roast 45 minutes, rotating peppers every 10–15 minutes to make sure all sides are charred. After roasting, transfer peppers to a large bowl, cover with a kitchen towel, let steam 15 minutes, and then peel off skin.

1. Turn pressure cooker on to Sauté function and add ghee. When ghee is hot, add onions, peppers, and garlic and sauté until softened, about 4 minutes.

2. Add remaining ingredients, stir to mix well, and close lid. Choose Manual function and cook on high pressure 15 minutes. Allow pressure to release naturally.

3. When pressure is released, open lid and remove chicken. Roughly chop chicken and set aside.

4. Use an immersion blender to purée broth mixture. Return chicken to pot and stir.

5. Allow to cool and then divide evenly among six airtight containers. Store in the refrigerator until ready to eat.

PER SERVING   Calories: 234 | Fat: 10 g | Protein: 26 g | Sodium: 547 mg | Fiber: 2 g | Carbohydrates: 10 g | Sugar: 4 g

Asparagus Soup

This asparagus soup is a low-carb take on the classic split pea soup. Instead of using diced ham, you can use a ham bone to get that salty, meaty flavor. If you go this route, make sure to remove the ham bone before blending. This soup will last up to 1 week in the refrigerator.

INGREDIENTS | SERVES 6

2 tablespoons ghee

4 cloves garlic, minced

1 medium yellow onion, peeled and diced

1 stalk celery, diced

1 cup diced no-sugar-added ham

2 pounds asparagus, ends trimmed and cut in half

4½ cups no-sugar-added chicken broth

¼ teaspoon dried oregano

¼ teaspoon dried marjoram

½ teaspoon salt

¼ teaspoon freshly ground black pepper

1. Turn pressure cooker on to Sauté function and add ghee to pot. Once it's hot, add garlic, onion, and celery and sauté until softened, about 4 minutes. Add remaining ingredients and stir.

2. Close lid, turn pot to Soup setting, and set for 40 minutes. Allow pressure to release naturally.

3. Once pressure is released, use an immersion blender to blend ingredients together. If you don't have an immersion blender, you can transfer ingredients to a high-speed blender or food processor instead.

4. Divide soup evenly among six airtight containers and store in the refrigerator until ready to eat.

PER SERVING   Calories: 146 | Fat: 7.5 g | Protein: 12 g | Sodium: 558 mg | Fiber: 3.5 g | Carbohydrates: 11 g | Sugar: 4 g

CHAPTER 14

Freezer Meals

Beef and Cauliflower Bake

If you have Cauliflower "Rice" (Chapter 13) on hand, you can use 1½–2 cups in place of the cauliflower florets in this recipe. Just line the baking dish with the rice and continue with the recipe as written. This will keep in the freezer up to 3 months.

INGREDIENTS | SERVES 6

½ cup water

1 large head cauliflower, cut into florets

1 tablespoon olive oil

1 large yellow onion, peeled and diced

2 stalks celery, diced

1½ pounds ground beef

1 teaspoon cumin

1 teaspoon paprika

½ teaspoon salt

½ teaspoon freshly ground black pepper

2 tablespoons tomato paste

1 cup no-sugar-added chicken broth

1 cup full-fat coconut milk

1 large egg

2 cups shredded sharp Cheddar cheese

1. Combine water and cauliflower in a medium saucepan and steam until softened but not fully cooked, about 4 minutes. Remove from heat and set aside.

2. Heat olive oil in a medium skillet over medium heat. Add onion and celery and cook until softened, about 4 minutes. Add beef, spices, and tomato paste and cook until no longer pink, about 7 minutes.

3. Spread cooked cauliflower out in a 9" × 13" baking dish. Spread meat out evenly on top.

4. Combine chicken broth, coconut milk, and egg in a medium bowl and whisk to combine. Pour mixture evenly over meat. Sprinkle cheese on top and cover.

5. Freeze until ready to cook, up to 3 months.

6. Heating instructions: Bake in a 375°F oven 60 minutes or until hot and bubbly. Uncover and bake 5 more minutes or until cheese starts to brown.

7. Divide into six equal portions and store each portion in a separate airtight container in the refrigerator until ready to eat, up to 1 week.

PER SERVING   Calories: 533 | Fat: 37 g | Protein: 38 g | Sodium: 671 mg | Fiber: 3 g | Carbohydrates: 11 g | Sugar: 4 g

Taco Chicken

If you like your taco chicken spicy, you can crank up the heat by adding ⅛ teaspoon cayenne pepper to the spice blend before coating your chicken. This dish will freeze up to 3 months.

INGREDIENTS | SERVES 6

1 tablespoon chili powder

1½ teaspoons cumin

½ teaspoon paprika

1 teaspoon salt

1 teaspoon freshly ground black pepper

¼ teaspoon crushed red pepper flakes

¼ teaspoon dried oregano

¼ teaspoon granulated garlic

¼ teaspoon granulated onion

1½ pounds boneless, skinless chicken breasts

2 cups no-sugar-added salsa

1 (6-ounce) can green chilies

Green versus Red Peppers

Green chili peppers are those that have been picked before they fully ripen. Red peppers are green peppers that have been left on the plant to ripen. Typically, green chili peppers are spicier than red peppers and have a more potent flavor.

1. Combine spices in a medium bowl and stir to mix well. Add chicken to bowl and turn to coat each side.

2. Add coated chicken, salsa, and green chilies to a gallon-sized freezer bag. Freeze until ready to cook, up to 3 months.

3. Heating instructions: Allow chicken to thaw in refrigerator overnight. Transfer to slow cooker and cook on high 4 hours or until chicken is cooked through.

4. Divide into six equal portions and store each portion in a separate airtight container in the refrigerator until ready to eat, up to 1 week.

PER SERVING   Calories: 175 | Fat: 3 g | Protein: 27 g | Sodium: 1,027 mg | Fiber: 2.5 g | Carbohydrates: 10 g | Sugar: 5 g

Bacon Sausage Balls

These Bacon Sausage Balls are the perfect protein addition to any meal—breakfast through dinner. They also make a great low-carb snack if you need a protein-filled pick-me-up during the day. These balls can be stored in the freezer up to 3 months.

INGREDIENTS | SERVES 6 (MAKES 12 MEATBALLS)

4 strips thick-cut no-sugar-added bacon, chopped

½ medium white onion, diced

2 teaspoons dried sage

1 tablespoon coconut aminos

1½ teaspoons apple cider vinegar

1 tablespoon fresh chopped basil

1 teaspoon salt

½ teaspoon freshly ground black pepper

¼ teaspoon crushed red pepper flakes

1 large egg

1½ pounds ground pork

Precooking the Bacon

If you prefer some added crispiness, you can partially precook the bacon before adding it to the food processor. Lay strips on a baking sheet, cook in a 400°F oven 5 minutes, remove, and transfer to a paper towel–lined plate. Let some of the grease soak into the paper towel before chopping.

1. Combine all ingredients except egg and pork in bowl of food processor. Pulse until everything is finely chopped.

2. Transfer ingredients to a medium bowl and add egg and pork. Mix with your hands until everything is evenly incorporated.

3. Form into twelve balls and line in a single layer on a baking sheet. Freeze 4 hours, transfer to a gallon-sized bag or an airtight container and store in the freezer until ready to use, up to 3 months.

4. Heating instructions: When it comes time to cook, take balls out of freezer, line on a baking sheet, and cook in a 350°F oven 30 minutes.

5. Divide into six equal portions and store each portion in a separate airtight container in the refrigerator until ready to eat, up to 1 week.

PER SERVING Calories: 388 | Fat: 31 g | Protein: 22 g | Sodium: 687 mg | Fiber: 0 g | Carbohydrates: 1 g | Sugar: 0 g

Chicken and Broccoli Bake

This recipe is designed as a freezer meal, but if you want to bake it right away as part of your meal prep, that's okay too. All you have to do is bake it 45 minutes or until cheese is hot and bubbly, allow to cool, and then transfer to your meal prep containers. This dish will freeze up to 3 months.

INGREDIENTS | SERVES 6

1½ pounds boneless, skinless chicken breasts, cut into 1" cubes

1 cup broccoli florets

1 cup cauliflower florets

½ cup chopped cooked no-sugar-added bacon

¼ cup chopped white onion

2 cups shredded Cheddar cheese, divided

1 teaspoon salt

½ teaspoon freshly ground black pepper

½ teaspoon granulated garlic

½ teaspoon granulated onion

1 cup heavy cream

1. Combine chicken, broccoli, cauliflower, bacon, onion, and 1 cup Cheddar cheese in a large bowl. Toss to combine. Sprinkle spices on top and toss to coat.

2. Transfer chicken mixture to an 8" × 8" dish and spread out evenly. Pour heavy cream evenly over mixture. Sprinkle remaining cheese on top and cover with foil. Freeze up to 3 months.

3. Heating instructions: When it comes time to cook, bake covered casserole in a 350°F oven 1 hour. Remove foil and cook an additional 5 minutes or until cheese is starting to brown.

4. Divide into six equal portions and store each portion in a separate airtight container in the refrigerator until ready to eat, up to 1 week.

PER SERVING Calories: 474 | Fat: 33 g | Protein: 37 g | Sodium: 757 mg | Fiber: 1 g | Carbohydrates: 4 g | Sugar: 2 g

Chocolate Strawberry Smoothie Packs

These smoothie packs make blending up a fresh smoothie every morning extremely convenient. By measuring out all your ingredients in advance, you can have a high-protein, low-carbohydrate smoothie in under 30 seconds. These packs can be frozen up to 6 months.

INGREDIENTS | SERVES 6

1 large avocado, peeled, cut in half, and each half cut into three equal portions

3 cups frozen strawberries

6 tablespoons no-sugar-added almond butter

3 cups baby spinach

6 teaspoons chia seeds

6 scoops low-carb chocolate protein powder

1. In each of six sandwich bags, combine 1 piece avocado, ½ cup strawberries, 1 tablespoon almond butter, ½ cup spinach, 1 teaspoon chia seeds, and 1 scoop protein powder. Seal bags and store in freezer until ready to use, up to 6 months.

2. Preparation instructions: To make smoothie, add contents of sandwich bag to a blender with 1 cup almond milk. Blend and serve.

PER SERVING   Calories: 204 | Fat: 10 g | Protein: 15 g | Sodium: 82 mg | Fiber: 5 g | Carbohydrates: 17 g | Sugar: 7 g

Shrimp and Veggie Stir-Fry

Save even more time on your meal prep by purchasing a 12-ounce bag of frozen stir-fry or Asian medley vegetables and using those instead. Just make sure all vegetables in the bag are low-carb. Carrots and baby corn, for example, aren't low-carb friendly. This dish can be frozen up to 3 months.

INGREDIENTS | SERVES 6

1½ pounds mini shrimp, peeled and deveined

2 cups broccoli florets

1 medium green bell pepper, seeded and diced

2 cloves garlic, minced

1 teaspoon fresh minced ginger

½ cup coconut aminos

¼ teaspoon crushed red pepper flakes

¼ teaspoon granulated garlic

2 tablespoons avocado oil

1. Combine all ingredients except avocado oil in a gallon-sized freezer bag and massage bag to make sure everything is coated and evenly distributed. Store in the freezer until you're ready to cook, up to 3 months.

2. Heating instructions: Heat 2 tablespoons avocado oil in a wok or medium skillet, add contents of bag, and cook 7 minutes. Divide into six equal portions and store in airtight containers in the refrigerator until ready to eat, up to 3 days.

PER SERVING   Calories: 67 | Fat: 2 g | Protein: 12 g | Sodium: 633 mg | Fiber: 1 g | Carbohydrates: 6 g | Sugar: 2 g

Taco Casserole

If you want to bake this casserole immediately instead of freezing it, follow the directions as written but bake only 25 minutes or until cheese is bubbly and starting to brown. Otherwise, this will keep in the freezer up to 3 months.

INGREDIENTS | SERVES 6

1 tablespoon olive oil

1 pound ground turkey

1 medium yellow onion, peeled and chopped

1 tablespoon chili powder

1½ teaspoons cumin

½ teaspoon paprika

1 teaspoon salt

1 teaspoon freshly ground black pepper

¼ teaspoon oregano

¼ teaspoon crushed red pepper flakes

¼ teaspoon granulated garlic

¼ teaspoon granulated onion

1 large zucchini, shredded and strained

1 (14-ounce) can diced fire-roasted tomatoes

1 (6-ounce) can green chilies

2 cups Cauliflower "Rice" (Chapter 13)

1 cup shredded Monterey jack cheese

1. Heat olive oil in a medium skillet over medium heat. Add ground turkey and onions. While turkey is cooking, add spices to skillet and continue cooking until turkey is no longer pink, about 7 minutes. Remove from heat and stir in zucchini, tomatoes, and chilies.

2. Spread Cauliflower "Rice" evenly on the bottom of a 9" × 13" pan. Pour turkey mixture on top and spread out evenly. Sprinkle cheese on top. Cover and store in the freezer until ready to bake, up to 3 months.

3. Heating instructions: Bake covered in a 350°F oven 1 hour. Remove foil and bake another 5–10 minutes or until cheese is bubbly and starts to brown. Divide into six equal portions and store in an airtight container in the refrigerator until ready to eat, up to 1 week.

PER SERVING   Calories: 390 | Fat: 27 g | Protein: 27 g | Sodium: 1,104 mg | Fiber: 2.5 g | Carbohydrates: 9 g | Sugar: 5 g

Lemon Walnut Pesto Chicken Bake

If you prefer to make a traditional pine nut pesto, you can replace the walnuts in this recipe with the same amount of pine nuts. You can also use avocado oil instead of olive oil. This chicken can be frozen up to 3 months.

INGREDIENTS | SERVES 6

2 cups fresh basil

⅓ cup chopped walnuts

½ cup grated Parmesan cheese

3 cloves garlic, minced

½ cup olive oil

1 teaspoon salt

½ teaspoon freshly ground black pepper

1½ pounds boneless, skinless chicken breasts

2 tablespoons lemon juice

The History of Pesto

The word *pesto* comes from the Genoese word *pesta*, which means "to pound or crush." Pesto originated in Italy and originally consisted of basil, pine nuts, garlic, Parmesan cheese, and olive oil. It's commonly used as a quick sauce for pasta, but it's delicious on chicken as well.

1. Combine basil and walnuts in a food processor and pulse until broken down and incorporated. Add Parmesan cheese and garlic and pulse a few more times. Scrape down the bowl.

2. Close lid and turn food processor on. Slowly pour in olive oil as food processor is running. Stop when necessary to scrape down the sides of the bowl. Add salt and pepper and pulse a couple of times.

3. Scoop pesto mixture in a large gallon-sized freezer bag. Add chicken and lemon juice. Seal tightly and shake to coat. Freeze until ready to eat, up to 3 months.

4. Heating instructions: Let chicken thaw in the refrigerator overnight. Transfer to a 9" × 13" baking dish, cover, and bake in a 375°F oven 30 minutes. If desired, remove from oven, uncover, and sprinkle ½ cup mozzarella cheese on top. Bake another 5 minutes or until cheese is bubbly and starts to brown.

5. Allow to cool, divide into six equal portions, put each portion in an airtight container, and store in the refrigerator until ready to eat, up to 1 week.

PER SERVING Calories: 376 | Fat: 27 g | Protein: 29 g | Sodium: 589 mg | Fiber: 0.5 g | Carbohydrates: 3 g | Sugar: 0 g

Chicken and Veggie Stir-Fry

This basic chicken and vegetable stir-fry is easily adaptable. You can make it with steak and any different combinations of low-carb vegetables that you like. It will freeze well up to 3 months.

INGREDIENTS | SERVES 6

1½ pounds boneless, skinless chicken breasts, cut into 1" cubes

1 cup broccoli florets

1 medium red bell pepper, seeded and diced

1 medium yellow bell pepper, seeded and diced

¼ cup no-sugar-added chicken broth

¼ cup coconut aminos

2 tablespoons sesame oil

2 tablespoons sesame seeds

1 teaspoon minced fresh gingerroot

2 teaspoons arrowroot powder

2 tablespoons avocado oil

1. Combine all ingredients except avocado oil in a gallon-sized freezer bag. Seal tightly and massage bag to coat and distribute evenly. Freeze until ready to cook, up to 3 months.

2. Heating instructions: Heat 2 tablespoons avocado oil in a wok or medium skillet. Add contents of bag and stir-fry until chicken is cooked through, about 8 minutes. Divide into six equal portions and store in separate airtight containers in the refrigerator until ready to eat, up to 1 week.

PER SERVING Calories: 217 | Fat: 9 g | Protein: 27 g | Sodium: 349 mg | Fiber: 2 g | Carbohydrates: 5 g | Sugar: 2 g

Blueberry Vanilla Smoothie Packs

You can boost the vanilla flavor in this recipe by throwing in a couple drops of pure vanilla extract right before blending. These packs will keep in the freezer up to 6 months.

INGREDIENTS | SERVES 6

1 large avocado, peeled, cut in half, and each half cut into three equal portions

3 cups frozen blueberries

3 cups baby kale

6 teaspoons hemp seeds

6 scoops low-carb vanilla protein powder

1. In each of six sandwich bags, combine 1 piece avocado, ½ cup blueberries, ½ cup baby kale, 1 teaspoon hemp seeds, and 1 scoop protein powder. Seal bags and store in freezer until ready to use, up to 6 months.

2. Preparation instructions: To make smoothie, add contents of sandwich bag to a blender with 1 cup almond milk. Blend and serve.

PER SERVING Calories: 163 | Fat: 7 g | Protein: 12 g | Sodium: 6 mg | Fiber: 6 g | Carbohydrates: 15 g | Sugar: 7 g

Cilantro Garlic Lime Chicken

This chicken is prepped and ready to freeze in under 5 minutes. If you make one of these freezer bags every time you meal prep, you'll be on the way to fully stocking your freezer with meals that you can cook up without any extra preparation. This chicken can be frozen up to 3 months.

INGREDIENTS | SERVES 6

3 tablespoons olive oil

Juice from 2 large limes, about 2 tablespoons

½ cup chopped cilantro

3 cloves garlic, minced

½ teaspoon salt

1½ pounds boneless, skinless chicken breasts

1. Combine all ingredients in a gallon-sized freezer bag and seal tightly. Massage bag carefully to mix ingredients and coat chicken. Store in the freezer until ready to cook, up to 3 months.

2. Heating instructions: Allow chicken to thaw in the refrigerator overnight. Transfer to a 9" × 13" baking dish. Bake in a 425°F oven 25 minutes or until chicken is cooked through.

3. Divide chicken evenly among six airtight containers and store in the refrigerator until ready to eat, up to 1 week.

PER SERVING   Calories: 196 | Fat: 10 g | Protein: 25 g | Sodium: 245 mg | Fiber: 0 g | Carbohydrates: 0.5 g | Sugar: 0 g

Turkey and Garden Veggie Soup

This recipe is written as a freezer meal so you can prep it and cook it later, but it also freezes well after cooking. You can cook the soup right after you prep, divide it into six containers, and then freeze those containers and eat each portion when you're ready. This soup will keep in the freezer up to 3 months.

INGREDIENTS | SERVES 6

2 large vine-ripened tomatoes, seeded and chopped

2 medium zucchini, diced

1 medium yellow squash, diced

1 large yellow onion, peeled and diced

1½ cups no-sugar-added marinara sauce

1½ pounds ground turkey

1 quart no-sugar-added chicken broth, reserved for cooking

1. Combine all ingredients except ground turkey and chicken broth in a gallon-sized freezer bag. Store in the freezer until ready to cook, up to 3 months.

2. Heating instructions: Allow vegetables to thaw in the refrigerator overnight. On the day of cooking, add contents of freezer bag, ground turkey, and 1 quart chicken broth to slow cooker. Cook 6 hours on low or until turkey is fully cooked.

3. Divide evenly into six airtight containers. Store in the refrigerator until ready to eat, up to 1 week.

PER SERVING   Calories: 243 | Fat: 10 g | Protein: 27 g | Sodium: 260 mg | Fiber: 2.5 g | Carbohydrates: 12 g | Sugar: 7 g

Ham and Turnip Soup

If you don't have a can of evaporated milk, you can replace it with heavy cream or half and half. If you use regular milk, which has a higher water content, you won't get the same creamy consistency. You can keep this in the freezer up to 3 months.

INGREDIENTS | SERVES 6

2 cups peeled and diced turnips

1 cup diced celery

1 cup diced red onion

5 cups no-sugar-added chicken broth

1 cup diced no-sugar-added ham

½ teaspoon dried rosemary

½ teaspoon freshly ground black pepper

1 cup evaporated milk

Evaporated Milk versus Condensed Milk

Make sure you're using evaporated milk and not sweetened condensed milk for this recipe. Evaporated milk is milk that has had about 60 percent of the water removed. Sweetened condensed milk is also milk with the majority of the water removed, but it also has a significant amount of sugar added to it.

1. Combine all ingredients except evaporated milk in a gallon-sized freezer bag and shake to combine. Pour milk into a sandwich-sized freezer bag, seal tightly, and place bag in gallon bag. Seal gallon bag.

2. Store in the freezer until ready to cook, up to 3 months.

3. Heating instructions: Put all ingredients except milk in the pot of a pressure cooker. Turn on Soup setting and set for 10 minutes. Allow pressure to release naturally. When pot is depressurized, open lid and stir in milk.

4. Divide into six equal portions and store in separate airtight containers in the refrigerator until ready to eat, up to 1 week.

PER SERVING Calories: 152 | Fat: 6 g | Protein: 12 g | Sodium: 448 mg | Fiber: 1.5 g | Carbohydrates: 13 g | Sugar: 7 g

Ginger Pork Tenderloin

Cooking frozen meat in the slow cooker is not recommended. Since the heat is low, there is a safety concern that it might not reach a high enough temperature to kill any harmful bacteria. You should allow some time to thaw out the pork in the refrigerator before cooking. This tenderloin will keep in the freezer up to 3 months.

INGREDIENTS | SERVES 6

¼ cup coconut aminos

½ cup olive oil

2 teaspoons fresh minced ginger

3 tablespoons steak seasoning

1 teaspoon garlic powder

2 pounds pork tenderloin

Homemade Steak Seasoning

There are many premade steak seasonings available, but if you want to make your own, combine 2 tablespoons paprika, 2 tablespoons black pepper, 2 tablespoons salt, 1 tablespoon granulated garlic, 1 tablespoon granulated onion, 1 tablespoon coriander, 1 tablespoon dill, 1 tablespoon red pepper flakes, and 1 teaspoon paprika in a small bowl. Stir to mix well. Store in an airtight container in a cool, dry place.

1. Combine all ingredients in a gallon-sized freezer bag. Seal tightly and massage to make sure ingredients are evenly distributed and pork is covered in marinade. Freeze until ready to cook, up to 3 months.

2. Heating instructions: Allow pork to thaw in refrigerator overnight. Transfer contents of freezer bag to a slow cooker and cook on low 6 hours.

3. Divide into six equal portions and store each portion in a separate airtight container in the refrigerator until ready to eat, up to 1 week.

PER SERVING Calories: 334 | Fat: 21 g | Protein: 32 g | Sodium: 369 mg | Fiber: 0 g | Carbohydrates: 3 g | Sugar: 0 g

Artichoke Chicken

If you're using jarred artichokes instead of canned artichokes for this recipe, check the ingredients list and make sure that the marinade doesn't contain any added sugar. This chicken can be frozen up to 3 months.

INGREDIENTS | SERVES 6

1½ pounds boneless, skinless chicken breasts

½ teaspoon salt

¼ teaspoon freshly ground black pepper

½ teaspoon granulated onion

1 (14-ounce) can artichoke hearts, roughly chopped

½ cup chopped spinach

¼ cup Basic Mayonnaise (Chapter 9)

3 tablespoons lemon juice

1 tablespoon lemon zest

½ cup shredded Parmesan cheese

3 cloves garlic, minced

Pump Up Your Potassium

Artichokes are a rich source of potassium—a mineral that can be lacking in an unbalanced low-carbohydrate diet. Potassium helps reduce blood pressure, lowers anxiety and stress, and improves brain function. One medium artichoke contains 475 milligrams of potassium—about 15 percent of your needs for the entire day.

1. Season chicken with salt, pepper, and granulated onion. In a small bowl, combine remaining ingredients and stir to mix well.

2. Transfer chicken and artichoke mixture to gallon-sized freezer bag and store until ready to cook, up to 3 months.

3. Heating instructions: Transfer prepared chicken to a 9" × 13" baking dish, cover, and bake in a 375°F oven 30 minutes or until chicken is cooked through.

4. Divide into six equal portions and store each portion in an airtight container in the refrigerator until ready to eat, up to 1 week.

PER SERVING   Calories: 213 | Fat: 11 g | Protein: 26 g | Sodium: 332 mg | Fiber: 0 g | Carbohydrates: 2 g | Sugar: 0 g

Parmesan Ranch Chicken

If you have the freezer space, consider doubling or even tripling this recipe. The prep takes less than 10 minutes, and you can have several weeks' worth of meals ready to go in your freezer. This dish can be frozen up to 3 months.

INGREDIENTS | SERVES 6

1 cup almond flour

½ cup grated Parmesan cheese

½ teaspoon granulated garlic

½ teaspoon granulated onion

½ teaspoon salt

¼ teaspoon freshly ground black pepper

1 cup Ranch Dressing (Chapter 9)

1½ pounds boneless, skinless chicken breasts

3 tablespoons ghee, melted

1. Combine almond flour, Parmesan cheese, garlic, onion, salt, and pepper in a small bowl. Put Ranch Dressing in another small bowl.

2. Coat each chicken breast in ranch dressing and then dip in almond flour mixture, turning to coat entire breast. Transfer coated chicken breast to gallon-sized freezer bag and freeze until ready to cook, up to 3 months.

3. Heating instructions: Allow chicken to thaw in refrigerator. Transfer thawed chicken to a 9" × 13" baking dish and drizzle melted ghee on top. Bake 30 minutes in a 400°F oven. Turn oven to broil and continue cooking 5 minutes.

4. Divide evenly into six portions and transfer each portion to an airtight container. Store in the refrigerator until ready to eat, up to 1 week.

PER SERVING Calories: 415 | Fat: 23 g | Protein: 30 g | Sodium: 755 mg | Fiber: 0.5 g | Carbohydrates: 19 g | Sugar: 2 g

Ranch Cheddar Burgers

Bacon Chipotle Ranch Dressing (Chapter 9) makes the perfect condiment for these burgers. Pair them with some Cheesy Cauliflower Tots (Chapter 10) and you've got a delicious—and simple— low-carb meal. You can store these uncooked burgers in the freezer up to 3 months.

INGREDIENTS | SERVES 6

¾ teaspoon dried dill

1 teaspoon granulated garlic

1 teaspoon granulated onion

1 teaspoon dried minced onion

½ teaspoon dried chives

½ teaspoon salt

½ teaspoon freshly ground black pepper

1 tablespoon dried parsley

1½ pounds ground beef

6 ounces sharp Cheddar cheese, finely cubed

Lighten It Up

If you want to lighten up the fat content a little bit, you can make these burgers with ground chicken or ground turkey or a combination of both. All three meats freeze well and taste great with the ranch-and-Cheddar combo.

1. Combine spices in a medium bowl and stir to mix well. Add meat and cubed cheese and mix with hands until ingredients are fully incorporated.

2. Divide meat mixture into six equal portions and shape into patties. Transfer to a baking sheet lined with parchment paper and freeze 1 hour. Put partially frozen patties in a gallon-sized freezer bag and store in the freezer until ready to cook, up to 3 months.

3. Heating instructions: Cook patties over medium-high heat on a grill, flipping once halfway through, for 8 minutes.

4. Store patties in separate airtight containers in the refrigerator until ready to eat, up to 1 week.

PER SERVING Calories: 310 | Fat: 20 g | Protein: 29 g | Sodium: 448 mg | Fiber: 0 g | Carbohydrates: 0 g | Sugar: 0 g

Tuscan Spaghetti Squash Casserole

This recipe calls for cooked spaghetti squash and cooked shredded chicken, both of which can be made quickly in your pressure cooker. When meal prepping, it's a good idea to have both these items on hand at all times, as they're used in several recipes. This casserole can be frozen up to 3 months.

INGREDIENTS | SERVES 6

3 tablespoons ghee

3 cloves garlic, minced

8 ounces cream cheese, cubed

2 cups full-fat coconut milk

½ cup sun-dried tomatoes

1 cup shredded Parmesan cheese

2 teaspoons dried basil

1 teaspoon salt

½ teaspoon freshly ground black pepper

3 cups cooked spaghetti squash

1 cup cooked shredded chicken

Are They Really Dried by the Sun?

Sun-dried tomatoes get their name from the fact that they are literally dried in sunlight. Typically, tomatoes are pretreated with salt and then left in the sun 4–10 days, where they lose most of their water content. The original purpose was to extend the shelf life, but they add a unique flavor and texture to any dish.

1. Melt ghee in a medium skillet over medium heat and add garlic. Cook until fragrant, about 3 minutes. Stir in cream cheese and continue stirring until smooth.

2. Whisk in coconut milk and then add sun-dried tomatoes, Parmesan cheese, basil, salt, and pepper. Stir until cheese is melted.

3. Add spaghetti squash and chicken to a 9" × 13" baking dish, pour sauce on top, and toss to incorporate ingredients and fully coat spaghetti squash. Cover and freeze until ready to cook, up to 3 months.

4. Heating instructions: Bake in a 350°F oven 40 minutes or until hot and bubbly.

5. Divide into six equal portions and store in refrigerator in separate airtight containers until ready to eat, up to 1 week.

PER SERVING   Calories: 429 | Fat: 37 g | Protein: 12 g | Sodium: 566 mg | Fiber: 3.5 g | Carbohydrates: 16 g | Sugar: 6 g

Pizza Casserole

This recipe does require a little extra preparation before you put it in the freezer, but the few extra minutes it takes to cook the beef and vegetables are worth the added flavor when you cook it out of the freezer. It will freeze for up to 3 months.

INGREDIENTS | SERVES 6

1 tablespoon olive oil
2 cloves garlic, minced
1 pound ground beef
½ pound no-sugar-added pork sausage
1 tablespoon Italian seasoning
½ cup chopped yellow onion
¾ cup chopped red bell pepper
¾ cup chopped green bell pepper
¾ cup sliced white mushrooms
½ cup chopped pepperoni
½ cup chopped black olives
2 cups no-sugar-added pizza sauce
2½ cups shredded mozzarella cheese
¼ cup shredded Parmesan cheese

1. Heat olive oil in a medium skillet over medium heat. Add garlic and cook until fragrant, about 2 minutes. Add beef, sausage, and Italian seasoning and cook until meat is no longer pink, about 7 minutes.

2. Add onions, peppers, and mushrooms and cook until softened, about 5 minutes.

3. Transfer meat mixture to a 9" × 13" baking dish and spread out evenly. Sprinkle pepperoni and black olives on top.

4. Pour pizza sauce over meat and sprinkle with mozzarella cheese and Parmesan cheese. Cover and store in the freezer until ready to cook, up to 3 months.

5. Heating instructions: Bake covered in a 425°F oven 35 minutes. Uncover and continue baking 5–10 more minutes or until cheese is bubbly and starting to brown.

6. Divide into six equal portions and transfer each portion to a separate airtight container. Store in the refrigerator until ready to eat, up to 1 week.

PER SERVING   Calories: 559 | Fat: 40 g | Protein: 38 g | Sodium: 884 mg | Fiber: 2 g | Carbohydrates: 10 g | Sugar: 5 g

Blue Cheese and Spinach Burgers

These burgers take about 5 minutes to prepare and give you all the convenience of commercially frozen burgers without any of the bad ingredients. You can double the batch to get ahead on stocking your freezer. These uncooked burgers will keep up to 3 months in the freezer.

INGREDIENTS | SERVES 6

¾ cup chopped spinach

3 cloves garlic, minced

1 teaspoon salt

½ teaspoon freshly ground black pepper

2 teaspoons dried minced onion

¼ cup crumbled blue cheese

1½ pounds ground beef

Swap the Cheese

If you're not a fan of the strong flavor of blue cheese, you can make a milder version of this burger by replacing it with crumbled feta cheese.

1. Combine all ingredients in a large bowl and mix until incorporated. Split beef mixture into six equal portions and form into patties. Lay patties out in a single layer on a baking sheet and freeze 1 hour.

2. After patties are partially frozen, transfer to gallon-sized freezer bag and freeze until ready to cook, up to 3 months.

3. Heating instructions: When ready to cook, heat over medium-high heat on a grill, turning once, until meat is cooked through, about 8 minutes.

4. Store each burger in a separate airtight container in the refrigerator until ready to eat, up to 1 week.

PER SERVING Calories: 220 | Fat: 12 g | Protein: 23 g | Sodium: 529 mg | Fiber: 0 g | Carbohydrates: 1 g | Sugar: 0 g

CHAPTER 15

Appetizers and Snacks

Coconut Yogurt

Once you make your own yogurt, you will never go back. This recipe does take some time, but when the yogurt is done, you'll have enough to last the whole week. You can even double the batch and freeze it for later, since cold temperatures will keep the probiotics alive.

INGREDIENTS | SERVES 6

3 (14-ounce) cans full-fat coconut milk

2 tablespoons unflavored grass-fed gelatin

3 probiotic capsules

Good Bugs

Probiotics are good bacteria that are similar to the bacteria that naturally live in your digestive tract. These bacteria don't just help keep you regular; they keep your gut, which affects your entire body, healthy. High heat and air can kill probiotics, so it's important to keep probiotic-rich foods cold.

1. Preheat oven to 110°F.

2. Heat coconut milk in a small saucepan over medium heat until it reaches a temperature of 180°F. (It's important that you use a thermometer for this, as this is a way to pasteurize the milk and prevent unwanted bacteria from forming.) Do not boil.

3. While coconut milk is hot, stir in gelatin until fully incorporated. Cover coconut milk and allow to cool to 100°F.

4. Transfer ½ cup of cooled coconut milk to a small bowl and open probiotic capsules into it. Stir well.

5. Combine coconut milk with probiotics with the remainder of the coconut milk, making sure to stir thoroughly. Pour coconut milk evenly into six glass jars with lids.

6. Place a baking sheet in the middle rack of your oven and place jars on sheet. Allow to sit in 110°F oven 8 hours.

7. Allow yogurt to cool, cover, and store in the refrigerator up to 1 week.

PER SERVING Calories: 417 | Fat: 41 g | Protein: 12 g | Sodium: 43 mg | Fiber: 0 g | Carbohydrates: 5 g | Sugar: 0 g

Chicken Nuggets

Who needs frozen chicken nuggets when you have this healthy version? These nuggets are ready in about 15 minutes. You can also freeze them and store them in the freezer up to 3 months.

INGREDIENTS | SERVES 6

2 large eggs

1 cup almond flour

½ teaspoon salt

¼ teaspoon freshly ground black pepper

½ teaspoon dried parsley flakes

1 pound chicken breasts, cut into nugget-sized pieces

Protein Packed Salad

These chicken nuggets make a nice addition to any of the Mason jar salads because they lend a nutty flavor and a little bit of texture. Just cook, roughly chop, and then replace the protein in the salad with the cooked nuggets.

1. Preheat oven to 450°F.

2. Beat eggs in a small mixing bowl. In a separate medium bowl, combine almond flour, salt, pepper, and parsley flakes.

3. Dip each piece of chicken into egg and then coat in almond flour mixture.

4. Arrange chicken nuggets in a single layer on a baking sheet lined with parchment paper. Bake 6 minutes, flip nuggets over, and then bake 6 more minutes or until golden brown and cooked through.

5. Divide chicken nuggets into six equal portions and store each portion in a separate airtight container in the refrigerator until ready to eat, up to 1 week.

PER SERVING   Calories: 208 | Fat: 4 g | Protein: 24 g | Sodium: 258 mg | Fiber: 0 g | Carbohydrates: 16 g | Sugar: 0 g

Peanut Butter Bars

These bars don't require any baking, so you can whip up a batch in under 10 minutes. It's best to store them in your refrigerator, but if you want to extend the shelf life, you can freeze them and let them thaw a little before eating. They will keep in the refrigerator up to 2 weeks.

INGREDIENTS | SERVES 6 (MAKES 12 BARS)

¾ cup almond flour

8 tablespoons ghee

¼ cup powdered erythritol

½ cup no-sugar-added creamy peanut butter

1 teaspoon vanilla extract

1. Mix all ingredients together in a medium bowl until combined.

2. Line an 8" × 8" baking pan with parchment paper and press mixture into pan.

3. Refrigerate 1–2 hours or until bars have hardened. Cut into twelve equal portions. Transfer to snack bags and store in the refrigerator until ready to eat.

PER SERVING Calories: 333 | Fat: 28 g | Protein: 6.5 g | Sodium: 91 mg | Fiber: 2 g | Carbohydrates: 16 g | Sugar: 2 g

Chicken and Zucchini Poppers

These poppers combine protein and vegetables, so they're good to include in your meal prep routine as a snack. They will keep you full until your next meal while also providing you with important nutrients and antioxidants. These poppers will keep in the refrigerator up to 1 week.

INGREDIENTS | SERVES 6 (4 POPPERS PER SERVING)

1½ pounds ground chicken

2 cups grated zucchini

2 medium scallions, chopped

½ teaspoon garlic powder

1 teaspoon salt

½ teaspoon freshly ground black pepper

2 tablespoons olive oil

1. Mix all ingredients except olive oil in a medium bowl. Divide mixture into twenty-four equal portions and form mixture into nuggets.

2. Heat olive oil in a medium skillet over medium heat. Cook each nugget 5 minutes on each side or until golden brown on the outside and cooked all the way through.

3. Divide cooked poppers into six servings and put each serving in an airtight container. Store in the refrigerator until ready to eat.

PER SERVING Calories: 296 | Fat: 23 g | Protein: 19 g | Sodium: 482 mg | Fiber: 0 g | Carbohydrates: 2 g | Sugar: 1 g

Buffalo Chicken Celery Boats

These celery boats are best served with Ranch Dressing (Chapter 9) or Creamy Blue Cheese Dressing (Chapter 9). These will keep up to 1 week in the refrigerator, but if you want to keep everything crisp, you can leave the filling separate from the celery stalks and fill right before you're ready to eat.

INGREDIENTS | SERVES 6

2 cups canned shredded chicken

3 tablespoons mayonnaise

¼ cup Frank's RedHot

¼ teaspoon salt

⅛ teaspoon freshly ground black pepper

12 stalks celery, cut into 4" pieces

1. Combine shredded chicken, mayonnaise, hot sauce, salt, and pepper in a medium mixing bowl.

2. Scoop mixture evenly into wells of celery stalks.

3. Store in an airtight container in the refrigerator.

PER SERVING Calories: 332 | Fat: 12 g | Protein: 47 g | Sodium: 407 mg | Fiber: 2 g | Carbohydrates: 4 g | Sugar: 2 g

The Power of Celery

Celery is a nutrient powerhouse. It's anti-inflammatory, antihypertensive (which means it can help keep blood pressure normal), and full of antioxidants. Celery is also rich in dietary fiber, boosting weight loss and contributing to healthy digestion.

Spinach and Artichoke Hummus

This hummus can be made in under 10 minutes, including the time it takes to steam the cauliflower. Although classified as a snack, it makes a great topping for your meals too. You can keep this hummus in the refrigerator up to 1 week.

INGREDIENTS | SERVES 6

½ pound steamed cauliflower

1 cup chopped artichoke hearts

½ cup steamed spinach, chopped

¼ cup Basic Mayonnaise (Chapter 9)

⅓ cup tahini

¼ cup fresh lemon juice

3 cloves garlic

1 tablespoon olive oil

½ teaspoon salt

¼ teaspoon freshly ground black pepper

1. Combine all ingredients in a food processor and process until smooth.

2. If mixture is too thick, add more oil until you reach your desired consistency.

3. Divide into six equal portions and store each portion in a separate airtight container in the refrigerator until ready to eat.

PER SERVING Calories: 182 | Fat: 17 g | Protein: 4 g | Sodium: 284 mg | Fiber: 2.5 g | Carbohydrates: 6 g | Sugar: 1 g

Salt and Vinegar Chicken Wings

These chicken wings take a little more time to prepare, but they're delicious cold right out of the refrigerator, so the time trade-off is well worth it. They'll keep in the refrigerator up to 1 week.

INGREDIENTS | SERVES 6

2 cups water

2 pounds chicken wings

1½ teaspoons baking powder

3 teaspoons salt, divided

½ teaspoon garlic powder, divided

½ teaspoon poultry seasoning

¼ cup white vinegar

3 tablespoons apple cider vinegar

½ teaspoon dried parsley

¼ teaspoon dried chives

¼ teaspoon dried dill

¼ teaspoon onion powder

1. Preheat oven to 425°F.

2. Fill a large stockpot with steamer basket insert with 2 cups of water. Bring water to a boil over high heat.

3. Add wings to steamer basket, reduce heat to medium, and cook covered 10 minutes. Remove wings from steamer basket and set on paper towels to remove excess moisture.

4. In a large mixing bowl, combine baking powder, 1 teaspoon salt, and ¼ teaspoon garlic powder. Add wings to baking powder mixture and toss to evenly coat.

5. Arrange chicken wings in a single layer on baking sheets. Roast 20 minutes, turn wings over, and then roast 20 minutes more or until browned and crispy.

6. While wings are cooking, combine remaining ingredients in a medium mixing bowl and stir until incorporated.

7. Remove wings from oven and add to bowl with vinegar mixture. Toss to coat.

8. Divide into six equal portions and store each portion in a separate airtight container in the refrigerator until ready to eat.

PER SERVING   Calories: 286 | Fat: 19 g | Protein: 26 g | Sodium: 1,210 mg | Fiber: 0 g | Carbohydrates: 0 g | Sugar: 0 g

Chocolate Cashew Fat Bombs

If you don't have a mini muffin tray, you can pour melted mixture into an 8" × 8" baking dish lined with parchment paper. Once the mixture is cooled, cut into twelve equal-sized pieces, and you're done! This will keep in the refrigerator up to 2 weeks or in the freezer for 2 months.

INGREDIENTS | SERVES 12

½ cup no-sugar-added cashew butter

½ cup coconut oil

3 tablespoons cacao powder

3 tablespoons full-fat coconut milk

4 drops liquid stevia

½ teaspoon vanilla extract

⅛ teaspoon salt

1. Line a 24-well mini muffin tray with cupcake liners.

2. Combine cashew butter and coconut oil in a small saucepan. Heat on low until melted and incorporated.

3. Remove from heat and add remaining ingredients. Stir until smooth.

4. Pour mixture evenly into mini muffin tray. Place tray in freezer 15 minutes or in the refrigerator 1 hour to harden. Divide into six equal portions and store each portion in a separate airtight container in the refrigerator until ready to eat.

PER SERVING   Calories: 115 | Fat: 12 g | Protein: 2 g | Sodium: 25 mg | Fiber: 0.5 g | Carbohydrates: 2 g | Sugar: 0.5 g

Buffalo Chicken Bites

This recipe is simple, but it requires you to marinate the chicken in buffalo sauce 8 hours before baking, so keep that in mind when designing your meal plan and making your cooking schedule. Store Buffalo Chicken Bites in the refrigerator up to 1 week.

INGREDIENTS | SERVES 6

1 pound boneless, skinless chicken breasts, cut into 1" cubes

½ cup Frank's RedHot

1. Combine chicken pieces and hot sauce in a medium bowl. Toss to combine. Allow to marinate in refrigerator 8 hours.

2. Preheat oven to 375°F.

3. Spread chicken out on a baking sheet and bake 20–25 minutes or until chicken is cooked through. Divide into six equal portions and store each portion in a separate airtight container in the refrigerator until ready to eat.

PER SERVING   Calories: 91 | Fat: 2 g | Protein: 16 g | Sodium: 33 mg | Fiber: 0 g | Carbohydrates: 0 g | Sugar: 0 g

Baked Meatballs

These baked meatballs are the perfect protein-rich snack, or you can combine a few with a cup of cooked spaghetti squash and some marinara sauce and make an easy, quick meal. These meatballs will keep in the refrigerator up to 1 week.

INGREDIENTS | SERVES 6 (MAKES 18 MEATBALLS)

1 pound 90/10 ground beef

¼ cup minced yellow onion

2 cloves garlic, minced

¼ cup crumbled feta cheese

1 large egg

1 tablespoon dried oregano

¼ teaspoon Italian seasoning

½ teaspoon salt

¼ teaspoon freshly ground black pepper

1. Preheat oven to 400°F.

2. Combine all ingredients in a medium bowl and mix with your hands until fully incorporated. Drop by rounded tablespoonfuls onto a baking sheet.

3. Bake 15 minutes, rotate meatballs, and bake 15 more minutes or until golden and cooked through. Put three meatballs in each of six separate airtight containers and keep in the refrigerator until ready to eat.

PER SERVING Calories: 165 | Fat: 10 g | Protein: 17 g | Sodium: 312 mg | Fiber: 0 g | Carbohydrates: 1.5 g | Sugar: 0.5 g

Jalapeño Popper Dip

It's best to reheat this dip slowly on the stove. Put it in a small saucepan and stir over low heat until heated through. You can also heat it up in the microwave in 15-second intervals, stirring between each interval to make sure it doesn't burn. This dip will keep in the refrigerator up to 1 week.

INGREDIENTS | SERVES 12

1 pound no-sugar-added bacon, cooked and roughly chopped

16 ounces cream cheese

½ cup Basic Mayonnaise (Chapter 9)

½ cup plain Greek yogurt

4 medium jalapeños, seeded and minced

1½ cups shredded Cheddar cheese

½ teaspoon onion powder

2 tablespoons hot chili sauce

1. Preheat oven to 350°F.

2. Combine all ingredients in a food processor and process until smooth. Pour mixture into a glass 9" pie plate.

3. Bake 25 minutes or until mixture starts to bubble. Allow to cool. Separate into six equal portions and store each portion in a separate airtight container. Store in the refrigerator until ready to eat.

PER SERVING Calories: 427 | Fat: 40 g | Protein: 11 g | Sodium: 584 mg | Fiber: 0 g | Carbohydrates: 4 g | Sugar: 3 g

Zucchini Pizza Bites

These pizza bites are delicious cold, but if you want to reheat them, line them on a baking sheet and broil 2–3 minutes in the oven. These bites will keep up to 1 week in the refrigerator.

INGREDIENTS | SERVES 6 (MAKES 24 BITES)

2 cups shredded zucchini

1 large egg

½ teaspoon dried oregano

½ teaspoon dried basil

½ teaspoon salt

¼ teaspoon freshly ground black pepper

¼ cup minced green bell pepper

1½ cups shredded mozzarella cheese

Shredding Your Zucchini

You can quickly shred zucchini with a cheese grater by hand or put a grater attachment on your food processor. There's no need to peel the zucchini either, as the skin contains most of the vegetable's vitamin C and fiber content, so you want to include it in your dishes whenever possible.

1. Preheat oven to 400°F. Spray a 24-well mini muffin pan with nonstick cooking spray.

2. Use a cheesecloth or paper towels to squeeze out as much excess moisture as you can from zucchini.

3. In a medium mixing bowl, combine zucchini, egg, oregano, basil, salt, pepper, and green pepper. Divide the mixture evenly among the 24 wells of the muffin pan.

4. Sprinkle mozzarella cheese evenly on top of each well.

5. Bake 15 minutes or until cheese just starts to turn golden brown. Allow to cool 10 minutes and then remove from pan. Divide into six equal portions and store each portion in a separate airtight container in the refrigerator until ready to eat.

PER SERVING Calories: 52 | Fat: 2 g | Protein: 5 g | Sodium: 96 mg | Fiber: 1 g | Carbohydrates: 4 g | Sugar: 2 g

Bunless Turkey Burger Bites

These bunless turkey burger bites are great on the go. Take some ketchup, mayonnaise, and mustard with you in your container and you'll have the perfect snack. These will keep in the refrigerator up to 1 week.

INGREDIENTS | SERVES 6 (MAKES 24 BITES)

1 pound ground turkey
½ teaspoon salt
¼ teaspoon onion powder
⅛ teaspoon freshly ground black pepper
½ teaspoon garlic powder
24 pickle rounds
12 cherry tomatoes, halved

1. Preheat oven to 400°F. Line a baking sheet with parchment paper.

2. Combine ground turkey, salt, onion powder, pepper, and garlic powder in a medium bowl. Spoon teaspoonfuls of mixture onto prepared baking sheet and shape into mini burger patties. Bake 15 minutes or until internal temperature of 165°F is reached.

3. Remove from oven and allow to cool.

4. Once cooled, slide each mini patty onto a toothpick. Add 1 pickle round and 1 tomato half to each toothpick. Divide into six equal portions and store each portion in a separate airtight container in the refrigerator until ready to eat.

PER SERVING Calories: 145 | Fat: 6 g | Protein: 15 g | Sodium: 376 mg | Fiber: 0 g | Carbohydrates: 8 g | Sugar: 6 g

Avocado Chips

These avocado chips are best eaten right out of the refrigerator without any reheating. You can enjoy them as a snack or use them to add a nice flavor and texture to any of your Mason jar salads. They'll keep in the refrigerator up to 1 week.

INGREDIENTS | SERVES 6

2 large ripe avocados, pitted and peeled
¾ teaspoon salt
⅛ teaspoon freshly ground black pepper
⅛ teaspoon cumin
1 cup grated Parmesan cheese

1. Preheat oven to 350°F. Line two baking sheets with parchment paper.

2. Put all ingredients in a food processor and process until just combined.

3. Drop mixture by teaspoonfuls onto prepared baking sheets. Flatten into thin, round shapes.

4. Bake 15 minutes or until golden brown. Remove from oven and allow to cool. Divide into six equal portions and store each portion in a separate airtight container in the refrigerator until ready to eat. Sprinkle with extra Parmesan before serving if desired.

PER SERVING Calories: 70 | Fat: 4 g | Protein: 5 g | Sodium: 591 mg | Fiber: 0 g | Carbohydrates: 2 g | Sugar: 0 g

Cloud Bread

Cloud bread gets its name from the fact that it's light and airy like a cloud. With only a few ingredients that you're likely to already have on hand, you can make this cloud bread quickly when you want to add a sandwich to your meal prep menu. This bread will keep in the refrigerator up to 1 week.

INGREDIENTS | SERVES 6 (MAKES 12 PIECES)

3 large eggs
3 tablespoons cream cheese
¼ teaspoon garlic powder
¼ teaspoon dried rosemary
¼ teaspoon baking powder

1. Preheat oven to 300°F. Line a baking sheet with parchment paper.

2. Separate eggs, putting egg yolks in one medium bowl and egg whites in another.

3. Add cream cheese, garlic powder, and rosemary to bowl with egg yolks and beat until combined.

4. Add baking powder to bowl with egg whites and use an electric mixer on high to beat egg whites until stiff peaks form, about 5 minutes. Do not skip this step or stop beating too early, or your bread won't form.

5. Slowly fold egg yolk mixture into egg whites, stirring just enough to combine but not enough to break apart egg whites.

6. Spoon mixture into twelve even-sized rounds on baking sheet. Bake 20 minutes and then turn oven to broil and continue cooking 1 more minute or until breads turn golden brown.

7. Remove from oven and allow to cool. Store in the refrigerator in an airtight container.

PER SERVING   Calories: 60 | Fat: 5 g | Protein: 4 g | Sodium: 61 mg | Fiber: 0 g | Carbohydrates: 0 g | Sugar: 0 g

Blackberry Fat Bombs

These bombs last up to 2 weeks in the refrigerator but can last months in the freezer. If you want to make extra, put some in an airtight container or freezer bag and store them in the freezer, thawing a few at a time when you're ready to eat them.

INGREDIENTS | SERVES 6

1 cup coconut oil
1 cup no-sugar-added coconut butter
¼ cup blackberries
¼ cup blueberries
½ teaspoon vanilla extract
¼ teaspoon liquid stevia
1 tablespoon lemon juice

1. Combine coconut oil and coconut butter in a small saucepan and heat over low heat until melted. Allow to cool.

2. Transfer coconut oil mixture to a food processor along with remaining ingredients and process until smooth.

3. Pour into an 8" × 8" baking pan lined with parchment paper and refrigerate 2 hours or until mixture has hardened. Cut into twelve squares. Divide into six equal portions and store each portion in a separate airtight container in the refrigerator until ready to eat.

PER SERVING   Calories: 642 | Fat: 72 g | Protein: 0 g | Sodium: 1 mg | Fiber: 0.5 g | Carbohydrates: 1.5 g | Sugar: 1 g

Almond Butter Bars

During the cooler months, you can store these bars at room temperature if you prefer them softer. Refrigeration doesn't increase the shelf life; it just helps them hold their shape better. They will keep up to 2 weeks in the refrigerator.

INGREDIENTS | SERVES 6 (MAKES 12 BARS)

¾ cup almond meal
¾ cup unsweetened shredded coconut
½ cup powdered erythritol
1 cup no-sugar-added almond butter
2 tablespoons coconut oil

1. Combine almond meal, shredded coconut, and erythritol in a medium mixing bowl. Set aside.

2. Add almond butter and coconut oil to a small saucepan and melt over low heat, stirring occasionally.

3. Once melted, pour almond butter mixture into almond meal mixture and stir until combined.

4. Spray an 8" × 8" baking pan with nonstick baking spray and press mixture into pan evenly.

5. Refrigerate 4 hours or until bars have set. Cut into twelve equal portions. Store in the refrigerator until ready to eat.

PER SERVING   Calories: 387 | Fat: 29 g | Protein: 11 g | Sodium: 184 mg | Fiber: 3 g | Carbohydrates: 38 g | Sugar: 5 g

Powdered versus Granulated

Powdered erythritol looks just like powdered sugar, whereas granulated erythritol looks like regular white sugar. If you don't have powdered erythritol, you can make it by processing granulated erythritol in the food processor or a blender with arrowroot starch until it forms a powder.

Baked Zucchini Chips

You can crisp up these zucchini crisps after storing them in your refrigerator by setting your oven to broil and broiling 2–3 minutes, flipping halfway through. Watch them closely, though, as the broiler cooks them quickly. These chips will keep in the refrigerator up to 1 week.

INGREDIENTS | SERVES 6

2 large zucchini, sliced into thin medallions using a mandoline slicer

1 teaspoon salt

1 teaspoon garlic salt

1. Preheat oven to 225°F.

2. Sprinkle salt on zucchini medallions and allow to sit 10 minutes to pull out excess moisture. Place zucchini medallions on paper towels and blot to remove any water that has beaded on the surface.

3. Spray two baking sheets with nonstick cooking spray. Arrange zucchini slices in a single layer on baking sheets. Sprinkle with garlic salt.

4. Bake 45 minutes or until zucchini starts to crisp.

5. Remove from oven and transfer to airtight containers. Divide into six equal portions and store each portion in a separate airtight container in the refrigerator until ready to eat.

PER SERVING Calories: 18 | Fat: 0 g | Protein: 1 g | Sodium: 783 mg | Fiber: 1 g | Carbohydrates: 3 g | Sugar: 2 g

No-Bake Protein Bars

These protein bars come together in minutes, but they do require you to let them set 4 hours in the refrigerator. It's a good idea to plan to make these the night before you want them. They'll last in the refrigerator up to 2 weeks.

INGREDIENTS | SERVES 6 (MAKES 12 SQUARES)

1 cup almonds

½ cup shelled sunflower seeds

½ cup shelled pumpkin seeds

½ cup ground flaxseed

½ cup unsweetened shredded coconut

1 tablespoon cocoa powder

½ cup no-sugar-added sunflower seed butter

¼ teaspoon salt

½ cup coconut oil

2 teaspoons vanilla extract

2 drops liquid stevia

1. Combine almonds, sunflower seeds, pumpkin seeds, ground flaxseed, shredded coconut, cocoa powder, sunflower seed butter, and salt in a food processor and process until a coarse powder forms.

2. Melt coconut oil in a small saucepan over low heat. Add melted coconut oil to food processor, along with vanilla extract and stevia. Process until a thick dough forms.

3. Press mixture into an 8" × 8" baking pan lined with parchment paper. Place in the refrigerator and allow to chill 4 hours or until hardened. Cut into twelve squares. Store in the refrigerator until ready to eat.

PER SERVING   Calories: 557 | Fat: 52 g | Protein: 15 g | Sodium: 104 mg | Fiber: 10 g | Carbohydrates: 16 g | Sugar: 2 g

Ground versus Whole Flaxseed

Always use ground flaxseed instead of whole flaxseed. Whole flaxseed contains a hard shell that the body is unable to break apart, so when you eat flaxseed whole, you're missing out on most of the nutrients. It's best to store flaxseed whole in your pantry and then grind it right before using it. This keeps the fats from going rancid and allows you to absorb all the nutrients.

Cheeseburger Dip

This cheeseburger dip tastes just like the real thing, but it's more portable and perfect for taking with you on the go. Serve hot or cold with raw zucchini slices. It'll keep up to 1 week in the refrigerator.

INGREDIENTS | SERVES 6

1 tablespoon olive oil
1 clove garlic, minced
1 small yellow onion, peeled and diced
1 pound 90/10 ground beef
1 teaspoon freshly ground black pepper
1 teaspoon garlic powder
1 teaspoon onion powder
¼ cup Basic Mayonnaise (Chapter 9)
4 ounces cream cheese, softened
1¼ cups shredded pepper jack cheese
1¼ cups shredded Cheddar cheese
3 tablespoons minced pickles

1. Preheat oven to 375°F.

2. Heat olive oil in a medium skillet over medium heat. Add garlic and onions and cook until translucent, about 4 minutes.

3. Add ground beef, black pepper, garlic powder, and onion powder and cook until no longer pink, about 6 minutes. Remove from heat, transfer meat to a medium mixing bowl, and allow to cool slightly.

4. Add mayonnaise, cream cheese, and shredded cheeses to meat and mix well. Transfer mixture to a 9" × 13" baking dish and bake 30 minutes or until mixture starts to bubble.

5. Remove from oven and garnish with pickles. Divide into six equal portions and store each portion in a separate airtight container in the refrigerator until ready to eat.

PER SERVING   Calories: 518 | Fat: 42 g | Protein: 29 g | Sodium: 547 mg | Fiber: 0 g | Carbohydrates: 5 g | Sugar: 2 g

CHAPTER 16

Desserts

Lemon Bars

Because ghee has the milk solids removed, you can store these bars at room temperature if you prefer them softer; however, they will hold their shape better in the refrigerator for up to 1 week.

INGREDIENTS | SERVES 6 (MAKES 12 BARS)

6 tablespoons plus ½ cup ghee, divided

2 cups almond flour

⅓ cup plus ½ cup granulated erythritol, divided

2 teaspoons plus 3 tablespoons lemon zest, divided

½ cup fresh lemon juice

6 large egg yolks

2 tablespoons grass-fed gelatin

Zest Carefully!

When getting the zest from a lemon, you want to make sure to only get the yellow part, so make sure to spin the lemon around frequently as you zest. The white part of the lemon, called the pith, has a bitter taste that you don't want in your dessert.

1. Preheat oven to 350°F.

2. Melt 6 tablespoons ghee in a small saucepan over medium heat. Stir in almond flour, ⅓ cup granulated erythritol, and 2 teaspoons lemon zest. Remove from heat and press mixture into an 8" × 8" baking pan lined with parchment paper.

3. Bake 10 minutes to set crust. Remove from oven and allow to cool.

4. Melt remaining ½ cup ghee in the saucepan over medium heat. Remove from heat and whisk in remaining ingredients except gelatin until mixture starts to thicken and curdle. Strain through a cheesecloth. Add gelatin and stir until smooth.

5. Pour lemon filling over prepared crust and spread out evenly. Bake 15 minutes or until set. Remove and allow to cool. Cut into twelve equal portions and place two bars into each of six separate airtight containers or small snack bags and store in the refrigerator until ready to eat.

PER SERVING   Calories: 505 | Fat: 34 g | Protein: 15 g | Sodium: 32 mg | Fiber: 1 g | Carbohydrates: 5 g | Sugar: 0 g

Almond Butter Cheesecake

Cheesecake freezes really well, so if you don't think you're going to finish all twelve slices of this decadent treat within 2 weeks, you can wrap slices in foil, place each wrapped slice in a freezer bag, and store in the freezer for up to 3 months.

INGREDIENTS | SERVES 12

1½ cups almond flour

⅓ cup cacao powder

¾ cup granulated erythritol, divided

5 tablespoons ghee, melted

24 ounces cream cheese, softened

1 teaspoon vanilla extract

1¼ cups no-sugar-added creamy almond butter

1. Combine almond flour, cacao powder, ¼ cup granulated erythritol, and melted ghee in a small bowl. Mix until incorporated and then press into the bottom of a 9" springform pan.

2. Mix remaining ingredients in a medium bowl and beat with an electric mixer until smooth. Scoop mixture over prepared crust.

3. Refrigerate for 4 hours or until firm. Cut into twelve slices and store each slice in an airtight container in the refrigerator up to 2 weeks.

PER SERVING Calories: 387 | Fat: 32 g | Protein: 9 g | Sodium: 205 mg | Fiber: 3 g | Carbohydrates: 20 g | Sugar: 2 g

Coconut Cookie Dough

Let's be honest: when making cookies, it's often the cookie dough that's the best part. This cookie dough contains no eggs, so you can eat it raw without any of the risk. Store in the refrigerator up to 1 week.

INGREDIENTS | SERVES 6 (MAKES 24 BALLS)

¾ cup full-fat coconut milk

¼ cup granulated erythritol

¾ cup coconut flour

½ cup ghee, melted

1 teaspoon vanilla extract

¼ teaspoon salt

¼ cup unsweetened shredded coconut

1. Combine all ingredients except the shredded coconut in a medium bowl and use a handheld electric mixer to blend. Once dough forms, stir in shredded coconut.

2. Scoop by tablespoonfuls onto baking sheet. Chill in refrigerator until hardened, about 1 hour. Store four balls in each of six airtight containers in the refrigerator.

PER SERVING Calories: 233 | Fat: 24 g | Protein: 2.5 g | Sodium: 100 mg | Fiber: 9 g | Carbohydrates: 18 g | Sugar: 0 g

Chocolate Tart

Many of the dessert recipes call for cacao powder, so it's beneficial to have some in your pantry, but if you don't or you can't find it easily, you can use unsweetened cocoa powder instead. Store in the refrigerator up to 1 week.

INGREDIENTS | SERVES 12

1 cup almond flour

¼ cup coconut flour

¼ cup plus 3 tablespoons raw cacao powder, divided

¼ cup plus 6 tablespoons powdered erythritol, divided

5 tablespoons (melted) plus ¼ cup ghee, divided

¾ cup full-fat coconut milk

¾ cup almond milk

3 ounces unsweetened dark baking chocolate

3 large eggs

Cacao versus Cocoa

Cacao and cocoa are similar, but different enough to matter. They both come from the cacao bean, true, but cacao is raw and unprocessed, whereas cocoa has been roasted at high temperatures. Raw cacao is defined as a superfood because it's high in antioxidants, phytochemicals, and flavonoids. The roasting required to turn cacao into cocoa destroys some of these compounds, making it less of a nutrient powerhouse.

1. Spray a 9" pie plate with nonstick baking spray.

2. In a small bowl, combine almond flour, coconut flour, ¼ cup cacao powder, and ¼ cup erythritol. Add 5 tablespoons melted ghee and stir to combine.

3. Press mixture into pie plate to form a crust and put in refrigerator to set.

4. Combine coconut milk, almond milk, and remaining ghee in a small saucepan and stir over medium heat. Bring to a boil and then remove from heat.

5. Put unsweetened chocolate, 3 tablespoons cacao powder, and 6 tablespoons erythritol in a food processor and process until combined. Pour in coconut milk mixture and process as you pour. Add eggs and process until smooth.

6. Scoop mousse onto prepared crust and spread evenly. Refrigerate until firm, about 1 hour.

7. Cut into twelve equal slices and place each slice in a separate airtight container. Each slice will last up to 1 week in the refrigerator. You can freeze extras, which will keep in the freezer up to 3 months.

PER SERVING   Calories: 196 | Fat: 14 g | Protein: 5 g | Sodium: 30 mg | Fiber: 4 g | Carbohydrates: 26 g | Sugar: 2 g

Strawberry Cheesecake

This strawberry cheesecake requires absolutely no cooking since it uses gelatin to set. When planning out your cooking for the week, you can make this first, so it's chilled and ready by the time you're done prepping everything else. Store in the refrigerator up to 1 week.

INGREDIENTS | SERVES 12

4 tablespoons ghee, melted

2 teaspoons plus 2 tablespoons granulated erythritol, divided

¼ cup unsweetened shredded coconut

1 cup almond meal

3 teaspoons grass-fed gelatin

2 cups boiling water

½ teaspoon vanilla extract

16 ounces cream cheese, softened

1 cup chopped fresh strawberries

½ cup sliced strawberries (optional)

Fresh or Frozen?

This recipe calls for fresh strawberries, but if you prefer, you can opt for frozen. Frozen fruits and vegetables can be easier to work with when you're meal prepping because they last longer. In many cases, frozen produce is also more nutrient-rich than fresh produce because it was frozen right after picking—a practice that helps preserve nutrients.

1. Combine melted ghee and 2 teaspoons erythritol in a small bowl. Add shredded coconut and almond meal and stir to combine. Press mixture into the bottom of a greased 9" pie plate. Refrigerate to set.

2. Put gelatin in a small bowl and stir in boiling water. Keep stirring until gelatin is dissolved. Add 2 tablespoons erythritol, vanilla extract, and cream cheese and beat with a handheld electric mixer until smooth.

3. Add chopped strawberries to a blender or food processor and blend until purée forms. Fold purée into cream cheese mixture.

4. Pour cream cheese mixture into prepared crust. Chill until set, about 2 hours.

5. Cut into twelve equal slices and transfer each slice to a separate airtight container. You can store cheesecake in the refrigerator up to 1 week or freeze extra slices up to 2 months. If desired, garnish with sliced strawberries before serving.

PER SERVING   Calories: 221 | Fat: 17 g | Protein: 6 g | Sodium: 142 mg | Fiber: 0.5 g | Carbohydrates: 13 g | Sugar: 2 g

Flourless Chocolate Cookies

Whisking the egg whites until they're fluffy is an important step in getting these cookies to come out right, so don't skip it to try to save time. These will keep up to 2 weeks at room temperature.

INGREDIENTS | SERVES 12 (MAKES 24 COOKIES)

1 cup unsweetened cacao powder
2½ cups powdered erythritol
2 teaspoons arrowroot starch
½ teaspoon salt
2 large egg whites
1 large egg
2 teaspoons vanilla extract

1. Preheat oven to 350°F. Line two baking sheets with parchment paper.

2. Combine cacao powder, erythritol, arrowroot starch, and salt in a medium mixing bowl.

3. In a separate medium bowl, whisk egg whites until fluffy. Add whole egg and continue to whisk. Whisk in vanilla extract.

4. Add egg mixture to cacao mixture and stir until combined. Mixture will be stiff.

5. Drop by rounded tablespoonfuls onto lined baking sheets. Bake 12 minutes. Remove from oven and allow to cool. Divide into twelve equal portions and store each portion in a separate airtight container or snack bag at room temperature. You can freeze any extras up to 2 months.

PER SERVING   Calories: 30 | Fat: 0.5 g | Protein: 1.5 g | Sodium: 15 mg | Fiber: 3 g | Carbohydrates: 48 g | Sugar: 4 g

Lemon Cheesecake Mousse

This recipe comes out best if you use fresh lemon juice, but if you're in a pinch, you can use bottled lemon juice instead. Keep in mind that some bottled lemon juice isn't real juice, so try to find one that is. You can keep this mousse up to 1 week in the refrigerator.

INGREDIENTS | SERVES 6

8 ounces cream cheese, softened
Juice from 2 large lemons, about ¼ cup
1 cup coconut cream
½ teaspoon liquid stevia
¼ teaspoon lemon extract
⅛ teaspoon salt

Another Variation

If you want a lighter, fluffier version of this mousse, you can swap out the cream cheese for mascarpone cheese. If you do, the fat and calorie content will be a little higher, while the carbohydrates will stay roughly the same.

1. Beat cream cheese in a medium mixing bowl. Add lemon juice and beat until smooth.

2. Add remaining ingredients and beat until just combined.

3. Split into six glass jars with lids. Store in the refrigerator.

PER SERVING Calories: 201 | Fat: 20 g | Protein: 3 g | Sodium: 189 mg | Fiber: 0 g | Carbohydrates: 2.5 g | Sugar: 1 g

Cashew Butter Mousse

You can use any nut or seed butter for this recipe, but cashew butter has a unique taste and texture that makes it really decadent. It's worth going the extra mile to try it as written at least once. This mousse will keep up to 1 week in the refrigerator.

INGREDIENTS | SERVES 6

8 ounces cream cheese, softened
¼ cup no-sugar-added creamy cashew butter
10 drops liquid stevia
1 teaspoon vanilla extract
1 cup heavy whipping cream, chilled

1. Combine all ingredients except whipping cream in a medium mixing bowl and beat until smooth. Set aside.

2. In a separate medium bowl, beat whipping cream until stiff peaks form. Fold whipped cream into cashew butter mixture and beat 1 minute or until a fluffy mousse forms.

3. Divide mousse into six equal portions and transfer to glass jars with lids. Store in the refrigerator.

PER SERVING Calories: 274 | Fat: 28 g | Protein: 3 g | Sodium: 151 mg | Fiber: 0 g | Carbohydrates: 3 g | Sugar: 2.5 g

Mint Chocolate Brownies

If you're not a fan of mint, you can make these classic chocolate brownies by replacing the peppermint extract with 1 teaspoon vanilla extract. These brownies will keep up to 1 week at room temperature.

INGREDIENTS | SERVES 6

½ cup chocolate chips (sweetened with stevia)

½ cup grass-fed butter

3 large eggs

¼ cup granulated erythritol

½ teaspoon peppermint extract

Finding the Right Chocolate Chip

This recipe requires some advance preparation because it's likely that you're not going to find stevia-sweetened chocolate chips in your local grocery store, and you'll have to order them online instead. Make sure you're prepared and order a few bags to keep in your pantry. Lily's Dark Chocolate Baking Chips are a good option.

1. Preheat oven to 350°F. Grease an 8" × 8" baking dish.

2. Combine chocolate chips and butter in a small saucepan. Heat over low heat until melted. Remove from heat immediately.

3. Combine remaining ingredients in a medium mixing bowl and beat until frothy. Pour chocolate mixture into egg mixture and beat until fully incorporated.

4. Pour mixture into prepared baking dish and bake 30 minutes or until toothpick inserted in center comes out clean.

5. Allow to cool completely and cut into six equal slices. Store each piece in an airtight container or snack bag. Store at room temperature.

PER SERVING Calories: 178 | Fat: 18 g | Protein: 3 g | Sodium: 37 mg | Fiber: 0 g | Carbohydrates: 9 g | Sugar: 0 g

Pumpkin Pie Bites

Make sure you're getting pure pumpkin purée and not pumpkin pie filling, which is loaded with sugar and will drastically change the carbohydrate count for this recipe. These Pumpkin Pie Bites are kept in the freezer and will keep up to 2 months.

INGREDIENTS | SERVES 6 (MAKES 12 PUMPKIN BITES)

2½ cups unsweetened, shredded coconut

½ cup coconut oil

½ teaspoon liquid stevia

¼ teaspoon coarse salt

¼ cup collagen powder

¾ cup pumpkin purée, room temperature

1 tablespoon pumpkin pie spice

½ teaspoon vanilla extract

1. Line 12 cups of a mini muffin tin with cupcake liners.

2. Combine shredded coconut, coconut oil, stevia, and salt in the bowl of a food processor. Process on high 5 minutes or until a smooth "butter" forms. You may have to stop the food processor and scrape sides of the bowl a few times.

3. Remove ¼ cup of coconut mixture and pour evenly into prepared muffin cups. Add remaining ingredients to coconut mixture in food processor and blend until smooth.

4. Scoop pumpkin mixture onto coconut mixture in muffin tins and spread out evenly.

5. Place muffin tin in freezer 1 hour or until set. Put two pumpkin bites in separate snack bags and store in the freezer until ready to eat.

PER SERVING Calories: 280 | Fat: 29 g | Protein: 1 g | Sodium: 104 mg | Fiber: 3 g | Carbohydrates: 6 g | Sugar: 2.5 g

Chocolate Pudding

If you don't have instant coffee, you can simply omit it from the recipe. The coffee brings out a richer chocolate flavor, but you can make a delicious chocolate pudding without it. Store pudding in the refrigerator up to 1 week.

INGREDIENTS | SERVES 6

3 cups full-fat coconut milk

⅓ cup unsweetened cacao powder

¼ cup granulated erythritol

2 teaspoons instant coffee

1 teaspoon vanilla extract

3 tablespoons grass-fed gelatin

⅓ cup water

Basic to Gourmet

This chocolate pudding is great on its own, but you can kick it up a notch by adding low-carbohydrate fruits like berries and some crunchy toppings like nuts or sunflower seeds to it. You can even combine this chocolate pudding with the Vanilla Mascarpone Parfait (see recipe in this chapter) to make a layered chocolate and vanilla parfait.

1. Combine coconut milk, cacao powder, erythritol, coffee, and vanilla extract in a small saucepan. Stir with a whisk over medium heat until combined and frothy.

2. In a small bowl, mix gelatin and water. Add to saucepan and whisk until gelatin is fully dissolved.

3. Transfer pudding mixture evenly to six glass jars with lids and refrigerate until set, about 1 hour. Store in the refrigerator until you're ready to eat.

PER SERVING Calories: 285 | Fat: 24 g | Protein: 14 g | Sodium: 44 mg | Fiber: 2 g | Carbohydrates: 16 g | Sugar: 3 g

Cinnamon Bites

This recipe can be made with any nut/seed butter and any nondairy milk you have on hand. It comes out delicious with peanut butter instead of sunflower seed butter and coconut milk instead of almond milk. These Cinnamon Bites will last in the refrigerator up to 1 week.

INGREDIENTS | SERVES 6 (MAKES 12 BITES)

½ cup no-sugar-added sunflower seed butter

2 teaspoons cinnamon, divided

3 tablespoons coconut flour

3 tablespoons almond milk

¼ cup plus 3 tablespoons erythritol, divided

½ teaspoon vanilla extract

¼ teaspoon salt

1. Combine sunflower seed butter, 1 teaspoon cinnamon, coconut flour, almond milk, ¼ cup erythritol, vanilla extract, and salt in a medium bowl. Mix until incorporated.

2. In a separate small bowl, combine remaining cinnamon and erythritol. Set aside.

3. Roll dough into 1" round balls. Drop each ball into cinnamon and erythritol mixture and toss to coat.

4. Transfer to a baking sheet lined with parchment paper and chill in the refrigerator 2 hours. Once cooled, place two cinnamon bites in each of six snack baggies and store in the refrigerator until ready to eat.

PER SERVING   Calories: 141 | Fat: 11 g | Protein: 5.5 g | Sodium: 191 mg | Fiber: 4 g | Carbohydrates: 22 g | Sugar: 2 g

Pistachio Fudge

This fudge holds up really well in both the refrigerator and the freezer, so don't be afraid to double the batch. This fudge will keep in the refrigerator up to 2 weeks.

INGREDIENTS | SERVES 12

9 tablespoons grass-fed butter, softened

4 ounces cream cheese, softened

3 tablespoons cacao powder

2 tablespoons granulated erythritol

1 teaspoon vanilla extract

½ cup shelled pistachio pieces

1. In a medium mixing bowl, beat butter and cream cheese together until smooth. Add cacao powder, erythritol, and vanilla extract and stir to combine. Fold in pistachio pieces.

2. Press evenly into an 8" × 8" baking dish lined with parchment paper. Place in the refrigerator and allow to chill 1 hour.

3. Remove and cut into twelve equal-sized pieces. Put each piece in a snack bag and store in the refrigerator until ready to eat.

PER SERVING   Calories: 141 | Fat: 14 g | Protein: 2 g | Sodium: 35 mg | Fiber: 1 g | Carbohydrates: 5 g | Sugar: 1.5 g

Vanilla Mascarpone Parfait

This recipe calls for sliced strawberries, but it can be paired with any of your favorite low-carb mix-ins, fresh or frozen! This can be refrigerated up to 1 week.

INGREDIENTS | SERVES 6

1 cup mascarpone cheese

1 cup coconut cream

¾ teaspoon liquid stevia

½ teaspoon vanilla extract

¾ cup sliced strawberries

1. Combine mascarpone, coconut cream, stevia, and vanilla extract in a medium mixing bowl. Beat until peaks start to form, about 2 minutes.

2. Place 1 tablespoon strawberries in the bottom of each of six glass jars with lids. Top strawberries with equal amounts of mascarpone mixture. Add 1 tablespoon strawberries to top of each jar. Cover and refrigerate until ready to eat.

PER SERVING Calories: 213 | Fat: 21 g | Protein: 3 g | Sodium: 146 mg | Fiber: 0 g | Carbohydrates: 4 g | Sugar: 2 g

Pumpkin Spice Pudding

If you want to spend even less time on meal prep, you can replace the cinnamon, ginger, nutmeg, and cloves with 1½ teaspoons of pumpkin pie spice. This pudding will keep in the refrigerator up to 1 week.

INGREDIENTS | SERVES 6

¼ cup water

1 tablespoon grass-fed gelatin

1 (14-ounce) can pumpkin purée

1 (14-ounce) can full-fat coconut milk

2 teaspoons vanilla extract

¼ teaspoon salt

1 teaspoon ground cinnamon

¼ teaspoon ground ginger

⅛ teaspoon ground nutmeg

⅛ teaspoon ground cloves

¼ cup granulated erythritol

1. In a small bowl, combine water and gelatin. Stir to get rid of clumps and set aside.

2. Combine remaining ingredients in a medium saucepan and stir over low heat until smooth and warmed through.

3. Remove from heat and stir in prepared gelatin. Transfer pudding mixture to six glass jars with lids and place in the refrigerator until set, about 1 hour. Store in refrigerator until ready to eat.

PER SERVING Calories: 172 | Fat: 14 g | Protein: 6 g | Sodium: 118 mg | Fiber: 2 g | Carbohydrates: 15 g | Sugar: 2 g

Sunflower Butter Chocolate Bars

Many store-bought sunflower butters are sweetened with cane sugar or honey, so if you're buying sunflower seed butter instead of making it, check the labels thoroughly. Any added sugar will throw off the carbohydrate count. These bars will keep in the refrigerator up to 2 weeks.

INGREDIENTS | SERVES 12

1¼ cup almond flour

6 ounces grass-fed butter

⅓ cup powdered erythritol

¾ cup no-sugar-added sunflower seed butter

¾ teaspoon vanilla extract

¾ cup chocolate chips (sweetened with stevia)

1. Combine all ingredients except chocolate chips in a medium bowl and beat until smooth. Press into an 8" × 8" baking dish lined with parchment paper.

2. Heat chocolate chips in a small saucepan over low heat. Stir constantly until chocolate is melted. Remove from heat and pour onto sunflower seed butter mixture immediately.

3. Spread chocolate out evenly on top. Allow to chill in the refrigerator 2 hours or until hardened.

4. Once hardened, remove from refrigerator and cut into twelve equal-sized bars. Transfer bars to snack bags and store in the refrigerator until ready to eat.

PER SERVING Calories: 230 | Fat: 17 g | Protein: 3 g | Sodium: 5 mg | Fiber: 2 g | Carbohydrates: 22 g | Sugar: 3.5 g

Peanut Butter Cookies

These peanut butter cookies require only three ingredients (yes, really!) and can be easily whipped up at any time. It's best to make them in single batches, rather than doubling or tripling the recipe. These can keep up to 1 week at room temperature.

INGREDIENTS | SERVES 6 (MAKES 12 COOKIES)

1 cup granulated erythritol
1 cup no-sugar-added peanut butter
1 large egg

1. Preheat oven to 350°F. Line a baking sheet with parchment paper.

2. Combine ingredients in a medium mixing bowl and beat until dough forms.

3. Using your hands, form 1" balls with the dough and place balls on prepared baking sheet. Use a fork to press a crisscross pattern in the top of each dough ball.

4. Bake 12 minutes or until cookies are slightly browned.

5. Remove from oven and allow to cool. Once cooled, put two cookies into each of six snack baggies. Store at room temperature.

PER SERVING Calories: 267 | Fat: 22 g | Protein: 10 g | Sodium: 193 mg | Fiber: 2 g | Carbohydrates: 41 g | Sugar: 4 g

Chocolate Coconut Clusters

You can store these chocolate coconut clusters in the refrigerator 2 weeks or the freezer 3 months. If you want to get ahead, double the batch, store some in the refrigerator for now, and store the rest in the freezer for later.

INGREDIENTS | SERVES 12 (MAKES 12 CLUSTERS)

⅔ cup unsweetened shredded coconut

¼ cup coconut cream

2 tablespoons unsalted grass-fed butter

3 tablespoons cacao powder

3 tablespoons erythritol

⅛ teaspoon salt

¼ cup no-sugar-added sunflower seed butter

Toasting the Coconut

Toasting the coconut brings out its rich, nutty flavor, but if you want to make these even more quickly, you can skip that step. Alternately, you can purchase coconut flakes that are already toasted for you.

1. Preheat oven to 350°F.

2. Spread shredded coconut out in a single layer on a baking sheet. Bake 5 minutes or until starting to slightly brown, flipping coconut over once during baking. Remove from oven and set aside.

3. Combine coconut cream, butter, cacao powder, erythritol, and salt in a small saucepan over medium heat. Stir and then bring to a simmer. Remove from heat and stir in sunflower seed butter until smooth.

4. Fold toasted coconut flakes into cacao mixture until incorporated.

5. Drop by tablespoonfuls onto a baking sheet lined with parchment paper. Place in the refrigerator until hardened, about 1 hour. Transfer clusters to an airtight container or individual snack bags and store in the refrigerator until ready to eat.

PER SERVING   Calories: 77 | Fat: 7 g | Protein: 1.5 g | Sodium: 49 mg | Fiber: 1 g | Carbohydrates: 6 g | Sugar: 1.5 g

Peanut Butter Fudge

This fudge can be made with your favorite nut or seed butter; it doesn't have to be peanut butter. If your nut or seed butter is unsalted, add a pinch of salt to the fudge mixture. Fudge will keep in the refrigerator up to 1 week or the freezer up to 2 months.

INGREDIENTS | SERVES 12

1 cup no-sugar-added creamy peanut butter

1 cup plus 3 tablespoons coconut oil, divided

¼ cup coconut milk

2 teaspoons liquid stevia

½ teaspoon vanilla extract

¼ cup unsweetened cacao powder

2 tablespoons granulated erythritol

1. Line an 8" × 8" baking pan with parchment paper.

2. Place peanut butter and 1 cup coconut oil into a small saucepan over low heat. Stir until combined. Add coconut milk, stevia, and vanilla extract and stir until smooth.

3. Pour mixture into prepared baking dish.

4. Put remaining coconut oil, cacao powder, and erythritol in a small saucepan and stir over low heat until combined. Drizzle cacao mixture over peanut butter mixture.

5. Drag a toothpick through mixture to create a swirl pattern. Refrigerate until hardened, about 2 hours.

6. Once fudge has hardened, cut into twelve equal-sized squares and transfer each square to a snack bag or airtight container. Store in the refrigerator until ready to eat.

PER SERVING   Calories: 331 | Fat: 33 g | Protein: 5 g | Sodium: 92 mg | Fiber: 2 g | Carbohydrates: 7 g | Sugar: 3 g

Snickerdoodle Cupcakes

It's been said that a muffin is a cupcake without frosting. That being said, these cupcakes can double up as a dessert or a breakfast option, so one batch can provide breakfast and dessert for 6 days.

INGREDIENTS | SERVES 12

1 cup unsalted grass-fed butter, softened

½ cup granulated erythritol

3 large eggs

2 teaspoons vanilla extract

¼ cup heavy cream

3 tablespoons water

⅓ cup coconut flour

1 cup almond flour

1 teaspoon baking powder

¼ teaspoon salt

2 teaspoons cinnamon

½ teaspoon nutmeg

¼ cup crushed walnuts

1. Preheat oven to 350°F. Line a 12-cup muffin pan with cupcake liners.

2. Beat softened butter in a medium bowl until light and fluffy. Add erythritol and continue beating until incorporated. Add eggs, vanilla, cream, and water and beat until smooth. Set aside.

3. In a separate medium bowl, combine remaining ingredients except walnuts. Fold dry ingredients into wet ingredients and stir until just combined. Fold in walnuts.

4. Fill muffin wells evenly and bake 20–25 minutes or until toothpick inserted in center comes out clean.

5. Once cooled, transfer each cupcake to an airtight container or snack bag and store at room temperature.

PER SERVING   Calories: 234 | Fat: 20 g | Protein: 4 g | Sodium: 111 mg | Fiber: 3 g | Carbohydrates: 19 g | Sugar: 0 g

CHAPTER 17

Weekend Gourmet Meals

Zucchini Lasagna

This zucchini lasagna takes some extra preparation, but it's perfect for the weekend when you have a little more time. To save time down the road, you can double the recipe and assemble two lasagnas at once—cooking one for now and saving one for later! This lasagna will keep up to 1 week in the refrigerator.

INGREDIENTS | SERVES 6

1 tablespoon olive oil

3 cloves garlic, minced

1 medium yellow onion, peeled and diced

1 pound ground beef

2 (14.5-ounce) cans no-sugar-added tomato sauce

1 (12-ounce) can tomato paste

1 tablespoon Italian seasoning

1 teaspoon dried oregano

1 teaspoon dried parsley

2 teaspoons salt, divided

1 teaspoon freshly ground black pepper

4 large zucchini, cut into thin slices with a mandoline

1 cup ricotta cheese

1 cup cottage cheese

½ cup grated Parmesan cheese

2 tablespoons chopped fresh parsley

2 large eggs, beaten

2 cups shredded mozzarella cheese

Choosing a Curd

Cottage cheese is available in large curd, medium curd, and small curd. In layman's terms, the curd refers to the size of the chunks that are in the cheese. When using cottage cheese in lasagna, it's best to go with small curd, as it will mix the best with the ricotta, and you won't even know it's there when eating the finished product.

1. Heat olive oil in a medium saucepan over medium heat. Add garlic and cook until fragrant, about 2 minutes. Add onion and cook until softened, about 4 minutes. Add beef and cook until no longer pink, about 7 minutes.

2. Add tomato sauce, tomato paste, Italian seasoning, oregano, parsley, 1 teaspoon salt, and pepper to the cooked meat and stir to combine. Reduce heat to low and allow to simmer 1 hour.

3. While sauce is simmering, sprinkle 1 teaspoon salt over zucchini slices and let sit 10 minutes.

4. Combine ricotta cheese, cottage cheese, Parmesan cheese, parsley, and eggs in a medium bowl and stir to mix well.

5. Layer ⅓ of the zucchini slices in the bottom of a 9" × 13" pan. Spread ½ the ricotta mixture over zucchini and then spread ⅓ of the sauce on top of that. Put down another layer of zucchini, using ½ of what's left. Top zucchini with the rest of the ricotta mixture, sprinkle 1 cup mozzarella cheese on top of that, and top with half the remaining sauce. Assemble one more layer using the rest of the zucchini slices topped with the rest of the sauce and sprinkled with the remaining mozzarella cheese.

6. Bake in oven 1 hour or until hot and bubbly with cheese slightly browned. Allow to cool.

7. Cut into six equal portions and transfer each portion to an airtight container. Store in the refrigerator until ready to eat.

PER SERVING Calories: 418 | Fat: 20 g | Protein: 32 g | Sodium: 1,239 mg | Fiber: 7 g | Carbohydrates: 20 g | Sugar: 18 g

Gorgonzola-Filled Chicken Breast

Cooking the shallots and the garlic for a few minutes before preparing the stuffing cuts down their sharpness a bit so they don't overpower the chicken. If you like the sharpness of garlic and raw onion, you can skip this step to save time. This dish will last up to 1 week in the refrigerator.

INGREDIENTS | SERVES 6

1 tablespoon butter

2 tablespoons minced shallots

2 cloves garlic, minced

¼ cup crumbled Gorgonzola cheese

¼ cup chopped fresh parsley

1 teaspoon salt, divided

1 teaspoon freshly ground black pepper, divided

6 (4-ounce) boneless, skinless chicken breasts

1 teaspoon garlic powder

1 teaspoon onion powder

1. Preheat oven to 375°F.

2. Heat butter in a medium skillet over medium heat. Add shallots and garlic and cook until softened, about 3 minutes. Transfer to medium bowl and add Gorgonzola, parsley, ½ teaspoon salt, and ½ teaspoon pepper. Stir ingredients to mix well.

3. Cut a slit into the thickest part of each chicken breast. Divide the gorgonzola mixture into six equal portions and stuff a portion into each chicken breast. Sprinkle remaining salt and pepper, garlic powder, and onion powder on each side of chicken breasts.

4. Transfer chicken to a 9" × 13" baking dish and bake 30 minutes or until chicken is no longer pink and juices run clear. Remove from oven and allow to cool.

5. Store each chicken breast in a separate airtight container in the refrigerator until ready to eat.

PER SERVING   Calories: 125 | Fat: 5 g | Protein: 17 g | Sodium: 487 mg | Fiber: 0 g | Carbohydrates: 1.5 g | Sugar: 0 g

Spaghetti Squash Pie

The flavors in this recipe get even better as it sits in the refrigerator; over the course of 1 week, the spaghetti squash will soak up some of the sauce. If you have extra sauce on hand, heat it up and pour it over your slice of this pie to add some moisture before eating. Store in the refrigerator up to 1 week.

INGREDIENTS | SERVES 6

3 cups cooked spaghetti squash

1 tablespoon olive oil

2 cloves garlic, minced

½ cup diced yellow onion

1 pound ground no-sugar-added turkey sausage

2 cups no-sugar-added pizza sauce

¾ cup chopped spinach

1 teaspoon dried basil

½ teaspoon dried oregano

½ teaspoon salt

¼ teaspoon freshly ground black pepper

2 large eggs, beaten

1 cup shredded mozzarella cheese

Making Your Own Turkey Sausage

If you can't find a turkey sausage that doesn't have any sugar or other undesirable ingredients, you can make your own by combining 1 teaspoon Italian seasoning, 1 teaspoon dried parsley, ¾ teaspoon black pepper, ¼ teaspoon fennel seed, ¼ teaspoon paprika, ½ teaspoon red pepper flakes, 1 teaspoon salt, 1½ teaspoons dried minced garlic, and ½ teaspoon dried minced onion. Add spice mixture to 1 pound of ground turkey before cooking.

1. Spread spaghetti squash out in a 9" × 13" pan.

2. Heat olive oil in a medium skillet over medium heat. Add garlic and cook until fragrant, about 2 minutes. Add onions and cook until softened, about 4 minutes. Add turkey sausage and cook until no longer pink, about 7 minutes.

3. Add pizza sauce, spinach, basil, oregano, salt, and pepper to skillet and cook until spinach is wilted and sauce is bubbly.

4. Pour sauce mixture over spaghetti squash and stir to coat. Add beaten eggs and stir to incorporate. Sprinkle cheese on top.

5. Bake until set and cheese is melted and golden brown, about 1 hour. Remove from oven and allow to cool.

6. Cut into six equal portions and transfer each portion to a separate airtight container. Store in the refrigerator until ready to eat.

PER SERVING Calories: 396 | Fat: 26 g | Protein: 24 g | Sodium: 966 mg | Fiber: 4 g | Carbohydrates: 14 g | Sugar: 6 g

Supreme Meatza

This dish gets even better as it sits in your refrigerator, so don't be afraid to make it a day or two before you're ready to eat it. It's delicious hot and cold— just like pizza! This will keep up to 1 week in the refrigerator.

INGREDIENTS | SERVES 6

1 teaspoon salt

1 teaspoon dried oregano

1 teaspoon garlic salt

1 teaspoon freshly ground black pepper

½ teaspoon red pepper flakes

1½ pounds ground beef

2 large eggs, beaten

¼ cup grated Parmesan cheese

1½ cups no-sugar-added pizza sauce

⅓ cup chopped red bell pepper

⅓ cup chopped green bell pepper

¼ cup sliced black olives

2 cups shredded mozzarella cheese

¼ cup chopped pepperoni

1. Preheat oven to 450°F.

2. Combine salt, oregano, garlic salt, pepper, and red pepper flakes in a small bowl and stir to mix well.

3. In a separate medium bowl, combine beef, eggs, and Parmesan cheese and mix well. Add spice mixture and mix to combine.

4. Press beef into a 9" × 13" baking pan, getting it as flat and even as you can. Bake 10 minutes. Drain excess grease.

5. Spread pizza sauce evenly on cooked meat and sprinkle on peppers and olives. Cover with cheese and add pepperoni on top.

6. Bake another 5 minutes and then turn oven to broil and broil 3–5 minutes or until cheese is bubbly and starting to brown.

7. Remove from oven and allow to cool. Cut into six equal portions and transfer each portion to an airtight container. Store in the refrigerator until ready to eat.

PER SERVING Calories: 406 | Fat: 26 g | Protein: 35 g | Sodium: 1,245 mg | Fiber: 1 g | Carbohydrates: 5 g | Sugar: 2.5 g

Beef Tenderloin with Mushroom Sauce

If you're eating a serving of this beef tenderloin right away, make sure to let the meat rest 10–15 minutes before slicing into it. This gives it a chance to reabsorb all its juices so that you don't lose all the flavor. This dish will keep 4 days in the refrigerator.

INGREDIENTS | SERVES 4

1 cup evaporated milk

4 teaspoons arrowroot powder

1 tablespoon olive oil

1 teaspoon salt, divided

½ teaspoon freshly ground black pepper, divided

1 cup sliced baby bella mushrooms, divided

2 tablespoons butter, divided

4 (4-ounce) beef tenderloin steaks

2 cloves garlic, minced

The Lean Beef Tenderloin

Beef tenderloin is one of the leanest cuts of meat, but the lack of fat doesn't allow a lot of room for overcooking. If you cook the meat too long, you'll get dry, tough meat, so pay extra attention to cooking times when preparing lean meats.

1. Combine evaporated milk, arrowroot powder, olive oil, ¼ teaspoon salt, ⅛ teaspoon pepper, and ½ cup sliced mushrooms in a blender or food processor and process until smooth. Set aside.

2. Heat 1 tablespoon butter in a large skillet over medium heat and add beef. Sprinkle with remaining salt and pepper. Cook 6 minutes on each side or until steaks reach desired level of doneness. Remove beef from pan and set aside.

3. Add remaining butter to skillet and add garlic. Cook until fragrant, about 2 minutes. Add remaining mushrooms to pan and cook until softened, about 3 minutes. Reduce heat to low, pour in cream sauce, and allow to simmer until sauce thickens, about 5 minutes.

4. Transfer steaks to separate airtight containers and pour equal amounts of sauce on top of each steak. Allow to cool, then cover and store in the refrigerator until ready to eat.

PER SERVING Calories: 458 | Fat: 34 g | Protein: 26 g | Sodium: 705 mg | Fiber: 0 g | Carbohydrates: 9 g | Sugar: 6 g

Stuffed Chicken Breast Wrapped in Bacon

Wrapping the chicken breast in bacon helps keep it moist during cooking and also during storage. When reheating, heat the chicken at 275°F in oven about 20 minutes and then broil 2 minutes to crisp up the bacon on the outside. This chicken will keep up to 1 week in the refrigerator.

INGREDIENTS | SERVES 4

¾ cup chopped spinach

¼ cup crumbled feta cheese

1 tablespoon minced shallots

1 teaspoon salt, divided

4 (4-ounce) boneless, skinless chicken breasts

1 teaspoon granulated garlic

1 teaspoon granulated onion

8 slices no-sugar-added bacon

1. Combine spinach, feta cheese, shallots, and ½ teaspoon salt in a small bowl and stir to mix well.

2. Use a paring knife to cut a slit into the thickest part of each chicken breast, then sprinkle remaining salt, granulated garlic, and granulated onion all over chicken breasts. Stuff equal amounts of spinach and feta mixture into each slit. Wrap each prepared chicken breast with two pieces of bacon and secure closed with a toothpick if necessary.

3. Arrange bacon-wrapped chicken in a 9" × 13" baking dish and bake 25 minutes or until chicken is cooked through and juices run clear.

4. Allow to cool and then transfer each chicken breast to a separate airtight container and store in the refrigerator until ready to eat.

PER SERVING Calories: 400 | Fat: 27 g | Protein: 34 g | Sodium: 992 mg | Fiber: 0 g | Carbohydrates: 3 g | Sugar: 1 g

Zucchini Latkes

These latkes are delicious chilled, but if you want to heat them up, add a small amount of coconut oil to a medium pan over high heat and allow latke to sit in oil about 1 minute on each side. These latkes will keep in the refrigerator up to 1 week.

INGREDIENTS | SERVES 4 (4 LATKES PER SERVING)

3 medium zucchini, shredded
1 teaspoon salt, divided
2 large eggs, beaten
2 small shallots, minced
¼ cup almond meal
1 teaspoon dried parsley
¼ teaspoon freshly ground black pepper
3 tablespoons coconut oil

Water-Rich Zucchini

Zucchini is 95 percent water, which means that eating it contributes to your daily water intake, but this also means it can get soggy when cooked. Sprinkling salt on shredded zucchini and letting it sit for 10 minutes helps draw out excess moisture so the zucchini crisps up better when cooking. This also helps extend the quality of the zucchini as it sits in your refrigerator because it prevents it from getting soggy too quickly.

1. Place shredded zucchini in a large bowl and sprinkle with ½ teaspoon salt. Let sit 10 minutes.

2. After 10 minutes, squeeze excess water from zucchini and transfer to a paper towel to absorb any remaining moisture.

3. Combine zucchini and remaining ingredients except oil in a medium bowl and stir to mix thoroughly.

4. Heat coconut oil in a medium skillet over medium heat. Transfer zucchini mixture by tablespoonfuls to hot oil and press down with a spatula to flatten. Cook each latke 3 minutes on each side or until golden brown. Remove from oil and place on a paper towel–lined plate.

5. Place four latkes into each of four airtight containers and store in the refrigerator until ready to eat.

PER SERVING   Calories: 183 | Fat: 13 g | Protein: 6 g | Sodium: 630 mg | Fiber: 2 g | Carbohydrates: 12 g | Sugar: 4 g

Prosciutto-Wrapped Asparagus

This is the perfect meal prep side because it's delicious both heated up and chilled. There's no need to heat it up; just eat it right out of the refrigerator. This dish will keep up to 1 week in the refrigerator.

INGREDIENTS | SERVES 4

6 cups water

⅛ teaspoon salt

16 spears fresh asparagus, trimmed

4 ounces cream cheese

1 tablespoon minced shallots

1 tablespoon chopped fresh chives

8 slices prosciutto

What Is Prosciutto?

Prosciutto, which means "ham" in Italian, is thinly-sliced pork that's been aged during a dry-curing process. Dry curing involves rubbing the meat with a mixture of salt and other spices and allowing to sit for 6 months to a year. Unlike bacon and pancetta, which must be cooked before eating, prosciutto is ready to eat.

1. Preheat oven to 375°F.

2. Fill a medium saucepan with water and salt. Bring to a boil and add the asparagus. Boil asparagus 2 minutes and then immediately transfer to an ice water bath to stop cooking. Set aside.

3. Combine cream cheese, shallots, and chives in a medium bowl and stir to mix well. Carefully spread cream cheese mixture on prosciutto slices. Gather blanched asparagus in bundles of two and wrap a prosciutto slice around each bundle.

4. Arrange wrapped bundles in a single layer on a baking sheet. Bake 15 minutes or until asparagus is tender.

5. Place two bundles into each of four separate airtight containers. Store in the refrigerator until ready to eat.

PER SERVING Calories: 343 | Fat: 30 g | Protein: 14 g | Sodium: 933 mg | Fiber: 1 g | Carbohydrates: 3.5 g | Sugar: 2.5 g

Dijon-Rubbed Salmon

To reheat this salmon, heat a little butter or ghee on medium heat in a medium skillet. Cook salmon for a few minutes on each side to heat through and crisp up coating. This dish will keep 3 to 4 days in the refrigerator.

INGREDIENTS | SERVES 4

3 tablespoons Dijon mustard
4 (4-ounce) salmon filets
¼ cup almond meal
¼ cup chopped cashews
1 tablespoon dried parsley
1 teaspoon salt
½ teaspoon freshly ground black pepper

1. Preheat oven to 400°F.

2. Coat all sides of each salmon filet in mustard.

3. In a medium bowl, combine almond meal, cashews, parsley, salt, and pepper and stir to combine. Coat salmon in mixture and transfer to a 9" × 13" baking dish.

4. Bake 12 minutes or until fish flakes easily with a fork.

5. Allow to cool and then transfer each filet to a separate airtight container. Store in the refrigerator until ready to eat.

PER SERVING Calories: 200 | Fat: 10 g | Protein: 20 g | Sodium: 777 mg | Fiber: 1 g | Carbohydrates: 7 g | Sugar: 0 g

Lemon Herb Salmon

The best way to reheat salmon is by slowly warming it in the oven. Place salmon in foil or a parchment paper bag and squeeze a small amount of lemon on top. Close foil or bag and heat in a 275°F oven 15 minutes or until warmed through. This dish will keep in the refrigerator 3 to 4 days.

INGREDIENTS | SERVES 4

2 tablespoons olive oil
4 (4-ounce) skinless salmon filets
2 cloves garlic, minced
1 teaspoon salt
1 medium lemon, cut into thin slices
2 sprigs fresh rosemary, cut into 4 pieces

1. Preheat oven to 400°F.

2. Brush olive oil over salmon and place salmon into 9" × 13" baking dish. Spread minced garlic on top of each salmon filet and sprinkle salt on top of garlic. Layer lemon slices and place a sprig of rosemary on each filet.

3. Bake 15 minutes or until fish flakes apart easily with a fork.

4. Allow to cool, transfer each filet to a separate airtight container, and store in the refrigerator until ready to eat.

PER SERVING Calories: 72 | Fat: 6 g | Protein: 5 g | Sodium: 464 mg | Fiber: 0 g | Carbohydrates: 0 g | Sugar: 0 g

Swiss Cheese and Asparagus Quiche

To make this recipe more portable during the week, follow the directions as written, but instead of assembling the ingredients in a pie plate, assemble them in muffin tins. You can grab these egg "muffins" as you head out the door or freeze them and thaw them individually for later. These will keep up to 1 week in the refrigerator.

INGREDIENTS | SERVES 6

1 pound asparagus, trimmed and cut into ½" pieces

3 cloves garlic, minced

1 tablespoon minced shallots

2 tablespoons olive oil

1 tablespoon Parmesan cheese

1½ cups shredded Swiss cheese, divided

6 slices no-sugar-added bacon, cooked and chopped

6 large eggs

½ cup coconut cream

¼ teaspoon ground nutmeg

1 teaspoon salt

½ teaspoon freshly ground black pepper

Using the Right Onion

There are several different types of onions available; sweet onions, red onions, white onions, yellow onions, and shallots are the most popular. Sweet onions are best for frying, whereas red onions are best for eating raw. White onions tend to have the spiciest flavor and the most crunch, whereas yellow onions are milder and are considered the best onion for cooking. Shallots have the mildest taste and are best in delicate dishes, like egg-based quiches.

1. Preheat oven to 425°F.

2. Combine asparagus, garlic, shallots, and olive oil in a medium bowl and toss to combine. Spread asparagus out on a baking sheet lined with parchment paper, scraping out all the oil and garlic. Sprinkle Parmesan cheese on top. Roast 12–15 minutes or until asparagus are tender yet still have some crispness.

3. Transfer roasted asparagus to a 9" pie plate and spread out evenly on bottom. Sprinkle 1 cup Swiss cheese on top of asparagus and add chopped bacon on top of cheese.

4. Whisk together eggs, coconut cream, nutmeg, salt, and pepper in a medium bowl. Pour on top of asparagus and bacon. Sprinkle remaining Swiss cheese on top.

5. Turn oven down to 375°F and bake 40 minutes or until eggs have set and cheese is bubbly and starting to brown.

6. Allow to cool, then cut into six equal portions and store each portion in an airtight container in the refrigerator until ready to eat.

PER SERVING Calories: 412 | Fat: 33 g | Protein: 21 g | Sodium: 687 mg | Fiber: 2 g | Carbohydrates: 6 g | Sugar: 2 g

Stuffed Italian Chicken

If you want to make this meal more portable and quicker for the weekdays, you can cube the chicken, season it, and cook it in a large skillet with the other ingredients. Everything will melt together, and you can eat it as is or enjoy it on top of some spaghetti squash. This dish will keep up to 1 week in the refrigerator.

INGREDIENTS | SERVES 4

½ cup chopped roasted red peppers

3 tablespoons grated Parmesan cheese

3 tablespoons chopped fresh chives

¼ cup shredded mozzarella cheese

½ teaspoon dried basil

½ teaspoon dried parsley

½ teaspoon dried oregano

4 (4-ounce) boneless, skinless chicken breasts

1 teaspoon salt

½ teaspoon freshly ground black pepper

½ teaspoon garlic powder

¼ teaspoon red pepper flakes

1. Preheat oven to 350°F.

2. Combine red peppers, Parmesan cheese, chives, mozzarella cheese, basil, parsley, and oregano in a medium bowl and stir to mix well. Set aside.

   Use a paring knife to cut a slit into the thickest part of each chicken breast. Scoop equal amounts of red pepper mixture into slit and secure chicken breasts closed with a toothpick. Arrange chicken in a single layer in a 9" × 13" baking dish.

3. Combine salt, pepper, garlic powder, and red pepper flakes in a small bowl and stir to mix well. Sprinkle over chicken.

4. Bake 20 minutes, then turn oven to broil and continue cooking another 5 minutes. Remove chicken from oven and allow to cool.

5. Transfer each chicken breast to a separate airtight container and store in the refrigerator until ready to eat.

PER SERVING Calories: 247 | Fat: 12 g | Protein: 28 g | Sodium: 768 mg | Fiber: 0.5 g | Carbohydrates: 3 g | Sugar: 1 g

Feta-Smothered Filet Mignon

If you want these steaks as part of your meal prep rotation, but you want a little variety without changing it up too much, you can swap the feta cheese for blue cheese or goat cheese, which will give the finished product distinctly different flavors. This will keep in the refrigerator up to 4 days.

INGREDIENTS | SERVES 4

4 (4-ounce) filet mignon steaks

1 teaspoon salt

1 teaspoon freshly ground black pepper

¼ cup olive oil

¼ cup balsamic vinegar

2 teaspoons dry mustard

2 teaspoons dried rosemary

2 tablespoons butter, divided

1 large yellow onion, peeled and cut into slices

4 ounces crumbled feta cheese

1. Sprinkle salt and pepper on each side of steaks. Combine olive oil, vinegar, dry mustard, and rosemary in a gallon-sized sealable bag. Add steaks to bag, seal, and massage to coat steak. Allow to sit in the refrigerator 1 hour.

2. Heat 1 tablespoon butter over medium heat in a large skillet and add onions. Cook until softened, about 4 minutes.

3. Transfer onions to a plate and add remaining butter to pan. Cook steaks in hot butter 5 minutes, flip each steak over, and cook another 5 minutes.

4. Pile equal portions of onions on top of steaks and add 1 ounce cheese to each steak. Cover skillet and allow steaks to cook until cheese melts.

5. Remove from heat and allow to rest 10 minutes.

6. Transfer each steak to a separate airtight container and store in the refrigerator until ready to eat.

PER SERVING Calories: 707 | Fat: 46 g | Protein: 30 g | Sodium: 943 mg | Fiber: 7 g | Carbohydrates: 43 g | Sugar: 21 g

Prosciutto-Wrapped Pesto Chicken

This recipe comes together in minutes but looks and tastes like you spent hours preparing it. To reheat, wrap chicken breasts in foil and bake in a 350°F oven 20 minutes. Remove foil and broil 2–3 minutes to crisp up prosciutto. This dish will keep up to 1 week in the refrigerator.

INGREDIENTS | SERVES 4

1 cup packed basil leaves

1 clove garlic

⅛ cup pine nuts

⅓ cup olive oil

¼ cup grated Parmesan cheese

¼ teaspoon salt

⅛ teaspoon freshly ground black pepper

4 (4-ounce) boneless, skinless chicken breasts

4 slices prosciutto

1. Preheat oven to 400°F.

2. Combine basil, garlic, pine nuts, olive oil, Parmesan cheese, salt, and pepper in a blender or food processor and process until smooth.

3. Spread ⅛ cup of mixture on each chicken breast and then wrap one slice of prosciutto around the breast, securing in place with a toothpick if necessary.

4. Bake 30 minutes or until prosciutto is crispy, chicken is cooked through, and juices run clear.

5. Store each chicken breast in an airtight container and refrigerate until ready to eat.

PER SERVING Calories: 360 | Fat: 25 g | Protein: 29 g | Sodium: 481 mg | Fiber: 0 g | Carbohydrates: 1.5 g | Sugar: 0 g

Shrimp-Stuffed Mushrooms

You can quickly reheat these mushrooms by turning your oven to broil and broiling them for 3–4 minutes. This will slightly crisp up the cheese and the mushroom. These will keep up to 4 days in the refrigerator.

INGREDIENTS | SERVES 4 (3 MUSHROOMS PER SERVING)

12 whole button mushrooms
¼ cup butter
3 cloves garlic, minced
¼ cup chopped white onion
¾ cup cooked baby shrimp
¼ cup shredded Italian-blend cheese

Italian-Blend Cheese

Many stores carry Italian-blend shredded cheeses, although the ingredients differ. Most are a combination of provolone, mozzarella, Parmesan, Romano and/or Asiago cheeses. If you don't have Italian-blend cheese, you can use any combination of these cheeses to create your own mixture.

1. Preheat oven to 325°F.

2. Remove stems from mushrooms and roughly chop.

3. Heat butter in a medium skillet over medium-high heat. Add garlic and cook until fragrant, about 2 minutes. Add onion and chopped mushroom stems and cook until soft, about 4 minutes.

4. Add shrimp and cook 1 minute just to warm up and incorporate flavors. Remove from heat. Scoop mixture into each mushroom cap and pour garlic butter sauce on top. Sprinkle with cheese.

5. Bake 10–15 minutes or until mushrooms soften and cheese is bubbly and starts to brown.

6. Transfer three mushrooms to each of four separate airtight containers and store in the refrigerator until ready to eat.

PER SERVING Calories: 207 | Fat: 19 g | Protein: 6 g | Sodium: 90 mg | Fiber: 1 g | Carbohydrates: 5 g | Sugar: 2 g

Red Pepper Chicken

The best way to reheat this red pepper chicken is to wrap each breast in aluminum foil and bake in a 300°F oven about 20 minutes or until chicken is hot. The low temperature and aluminum foil work together to keep the chicken moist. This dish will keep up to 1 week in the refrigerator.

INGREDIENTS | SERVES 4

4 (4-ounce) boneless, skinless chicken breasts

1 cup chopped roasted red peppers

½ cup crumbled feta cheese

1 cup almond meal

1 tablespoon dried parsley

½ teaspoon salt

¼ teaspoon freshly ground black pepper

¼ teaspoon granulated garlic

1 large egg, beaten

2 tablespoons ghee

Red Pepper Sauce

If you have a few extra minutes and want to add a quick red pepper sauce, combine 1 cup sour cream and ¼ cup roasted red peppers in a blender and blend until smooth. Transfer mixture to a medium saucepan and add ½ teaspoon salt, ¼ teaspoon pepper, and ¼ teaspoon garlic powder. Heat over medium heat and simmer 5 minutes. Pour sauce over chicken before storing or right before eating.

1. Pound each chicken breast with a mallet to flatten slightly. Using a paring knife, cut pockets into the thickest part of each chicken breast. Set aside.

2. In a small bowl, combine red peppers and feta cheese and stir to mix well. Stuff equal amounts of pepper mixture into the pocket of each chicken breast. Secure chicken breasts closed with toothpicks.

3. In a separate small bowl, combine almond meal, parsley, salt, pepper, and granulated garlic. Stir to mix well.

4. Dip each stuffed chicken breast in the beaten egg and then coat with almond meal mixture.

5. Heat ghee in a medium skillet over medium-high heat. Add chicken to skillet and cook 7 minutes, flip each breast over, and cook an additional 7 minutes or until chicken is cooked through and juices run clear.

6. Transfer each stuffed chicken breast to a separate airtight container and store in the refrigerator until ready to eat.

PER SERVING   Calories: 388 | Fat: 15 g | Protein: 33 g | Sodium: 536 mg | Fiber: 2 g | Carbohydrates: 28 g | Sugar: 3 g

Sausage-Stuffed Eggplant

To reheat this dish, bake it in a 350°F oven 15 minutes. Once eggplant is heated through, turn oven to broil and continue cooking 2 minutes to crisp up the cheese. This will keep up to 1 week in the refrigerator.

INGREDIENTS | SERVES 4

2 small eggplants, cut in half lengthwise

1 tablespoon olive oil

1 teaspoon salt

1 pound ground no-sugar-added Italian sausage

½ teaspoon granulated garlic

½ teaspoon Italian seasoning

¼ teaspoon dried oregano

¼ teaspoon freshly ground black pepper

¼ cup almond meal

3 cups no-sugar-added marinara sauce, divided

2 cups shredded mozzarella cheese, divided

¼ cup grated Parmesan cheese

2 large eggs, beaten

1. Preheat oven to 400°F.

2. Brush cut side of eggplants with olive oil and sprinkle with salt. Place on a baking sheet and roast 30 minutes. Remove from oven and allow to cool.

3. Cook sausage in a medium skillet over medium heat until no longer pink, about 8 minutes. Transfer to a medium bowl and add granulated garlic, Italian seasoning, oregano, pepper, almond meal, 1 cup marinara sauce, 1 cup mozzarella cheese, Parmesan cheese, and egg. Mix well until fully incorporated.

4. Scoop out the flesh of the roasted eggplant, leaving just enough so that the eggplant skin forms a shell. Chop the eggplant flesh and fold into sausage mixture, stirring to incorporate.

5. Scoop equal amounts of sausage and eggplant mixture into each eggplant half. Pour remaining marinara sauce on top and sprinkle with remaining mozzarella cheese.

6. Bake 20 minutes or until cheese is bubbly and starts to brown.

7. Transfer each eggplant half to a separate airtight container and store in the refrigerator until ready to eat.

PER SERVING Calories: 669 | Fat: 43 g | Protein: 38 g | Sodium: 1,862 mg | Fiber: 9 g | Carbohydrates: 28 g | Sugar: 14 g

Lemon Pepper Salmon

Fish isn't as popular as other protein sources for meal prepping because it doesn't last as long in the refrigerator. This dish will only last 3 days. This dish provides 4 servings instead of 6 so you can eat it while it's still good.

INGREDIENTS | SERVES 4

4 (4-ounce) salmon filets

2 teaspoons lemon pepper

1 teaspoon salt

3 tablespoons butter

2 cloves garlic, minced

2 tablespoons lemon juice

¼ cup water

1 (14-ounce) can petite diced tomatoes

½ cup chopped fresh parsley

Fresh Lemon Pepper

If a recipe calls for lemon pepper, and you don't have any on hand, but you do have fresh lemons, you can quickly make your own. Combine 1 tablespoon of lemon zest with 2 tablespoons of black pepper and 1 tablespoon of salt.

1. Season both sides of each salmon filet with lemon pepper and salt.

2. Heat butter over medium heat in a medium skillet and add garlic. Cook until fragrant, about 2 minutes.

3. Add salmon to the pan and pour lemon juice and water around it. Arrange tomatoes and parsley around salmon and cover skillet.

4. Cook 15 minutes or until fish flakes easily with a fork.

5. Transfer filets to separate airtight containers and scoop equal amounts of tomato mixture and sauce on top. Store in the refrigerator until ready to eat.

PER SERVING Calories: 254 | Fat: 16 g | Protein: 23 g | Sodium: 746 mg | Fiber: 2 g | Carbohydrates: 4 g | Sugar: 2 g

Swiss Mushroom Chicken

If prepping this meal in advance, you can leave the cheese off and add it to the chicken when reheating. You would heat the chicken in the oven, and once chicken is hot, sprinkle cheese on top and broil 3–4 minutes or until cheese is hot and bubbly. This chicken will keep up to 1 week in the refrigerator.

INGREDIENTS | SERVES 4

1 teaspoon granulated garlic

½ teaspoon salt

¼ teaspoon freshly ground black pepper

1 teaspoon dried basil

1 teaspoon dried parsley

½ teaspoon dried oregano

4 (4-ounce) boneless, skinless chicken breasts

2 tablespoons ghee

2 cloves garlic, minced

¼ cup chopped yellow onion

½ cup sliced white mushrooms

2 cups shredded Swiss cheese

1. Combine spices and herbs in a small bowl and stir to mix well. Coat chicken in dry rub, covering as much as possible, and set aside.

2. Heat ghee in a medium skillet over medium heat. Add garlic and cook until fragrant, about 2 minutes. Add onion and continue cooking until softened, about 4 minutes. Add mushrooms and cook until softened, another 4 minutes.

3. Add chicken to pan and cook 10 minutes on each side or until chicken is cooked through and juices run clear. When chicken is cooked, scoop mushroom and onion mixture onto each breast and top each breast with ½ cup cheese.

4. Cover skillet and continue cooking 5 more minutes or until cheese is melted.

5. Store each portion in an airtight container in the refrigerator until ready to eat.

PER SERVING Calories: 454 | Fat: 27 g | Protein: 43 g | Sodium: 389 mg | Fiber: 1 g | Carbohydrates: 6 g | Sugar: 1.5 g

Filet Mignon with Bacon Mushroom Cream Sauce

The best way to reheat filet mignon is by slow roasting it in the oven. When ready to eat, preheat oven or toaster oven to 250°F, wrap steak and sauce in foil, and heat about 40 minutes or until internal temperature reaches 110°F. You can keep this dish in the refrigerator up to 1 week.

INGREDIENTS | SERVES 4

1 tablespoon butter

4 medium shallots, diced

½ cup sliced baby bella mushrooms

3 slices cooked no-sugar-added bacon, chopped and patted dry

⅓ cup heavy cream

2 tablespoons sour cream

1 teaspoon salt

1 teaspoon freshly ground black pepper

4 (4-ounce) filet mignon steaks

1 tablespoon steak seasoning

1 tablespoon olive oil

Make Your Own Steak Seasoning

You can make your own basic steak seasoning by combining 2 tablespoons salt, 2 tablespoons smoked paprika, 1 tablespoon granulated onion, 1 tablespoon granulated garlic, 1 tablespoon dried oregano, 1 tablespoon coarse black pepper, and 1 tablespoon ground cumin. Use what you need and store the rest in an airtight container in a cool, dry place.

1. Preheat grill to medium-high heat.

2. Heat butter in a medium skillet over medium heat, add shallots and cook until softened, about 4 minutes. Add mushrooms and cook 3 more minutes. Add bacon to pan and stir in cream, sour cream, salt, and pepper.

3. Reduce heat to medium-low and allow to simmer until sauce thickens, about 5 minutes.

4. Coat each filet with steak seasoning, covering as much as possible, then brush olive oil over filets.

5. Cook filets on grill 5 minutes, then flip and continue cooking 4 minutes or until steaks reach desired level of doneness.

6. Remove steaks from grill and allow to rest 10 minutes. Pour equal amounts of cream sauce over each filet.

7. Store each portion in an airtight container in the refrigerator until ready to eat.

PER SERVING Calories: 505 | Fat: 43 g | Protein: 25 g | Sodium: 787 mg | Fiber: 0 g | Carbohydrates: 1.5 g | Sugar: 1 g

Two-Week Meal Plan

For this two-week meal plan, your cooking days fall on Sunday, Saturday, and Friday. If you are unable to cook on a Friday, you can cook a fresh breakfast Saturday morning, store the rest for the week, and then cook your remaining meals during the day on Saturday.

Monday
Breakfast: Bacon Spinach Egg Cups (Chapter 3)
Snack: Spinach and Artichoke Hummus (Chapter 15) with cucumber slices
Lunch: Bacon Turkey Burgers (Chapter 4) with Cheesy Cauliflower Tots (Chapter 10) and Ketchup (Chapter 9)
Dinner: Chicken and Mushroom Soup (Chapter 11)
Dessert: Chocolate Pudding (Chapter 16)

Tuesday
Breakfast: Bacon Spinach Egg Cups
Snack: Spinach and Artichoke Hummus with cucumber slices
Lunch: Bacon Turkey Burgers with Cheesy Cauliflower Tots and Ketchup
Dinner: Chicken and Mushroom Soup
Dessert: Chocolate Pudding

Wednesday
Breakfast: Bacon Spinach Egg Cups
Snack: Spinach and Artichoke Hummus with cucumber slices
Lunch: Bacon Turkey Burgers with Cheesy Cauliflower Tots and Ketchup
Dinner: Chicken and Mushroom Soup
Dessert: Chocolate Pudding

Thursday
Breakfast: Bacon Spinach Egg Cups
Snack: Spinach and Artichoke Hummus with cucumber slices
Lunch: Bacon Turkey Burgers with Cheesy Cauliflower Tots and Ketchup
Dinner: Chicken and Mushroom Soup
Dessert: Chocolate Pudding

Friday
Breakfast: Bacon Spinach Egg Cups
Snack: Spinach and Artichoke Hummus with cucumber slices
Lunch: Bacon Turkey Burgers with Cheesy Cauliflower Tots and Ketchup
Dinner: Chicken and Mushroom Soup
Dessert: Chocolate Pudding

Saturday
Breakfast: Bacon Spinach Egg Cups
Snack: Spinach and Artichoke Hummus with cucumber slices
Lunch: Bacon Turkey Burgers with Cheesy Cauliflower Tots and Ketchup
Dinner: Chicken and Mushroom Soup
Dessert: Chocolate Pudding

Sunday
Breakfast: Cauliflower Skillet Casserole (Chapter 3)
Snack: Peanut Butter Bars (Chapter 15)
Lunch: Spaghetti Squash Pie (Chapter 17)
Dinner: Beef Stir-Fry (Chapter 5) with Cauliflower Fried Rice (Chapter 7)
Dessert: Coconut Cookie Dough (Chapter 16)

Monday

Breakfast: Cauliflower Skillet Casserole
Snack: Peanut Butter Bars
Lunch: Spaghetti Squash Pie
Dinner: Beef Stir-Fry with Cauliflower Fried Rice
Dessert: Coconut Cookie Dough

Tuesday

Breakfast: Cauliflower Skillet Casserole
Snack: Peanut Butter Bars
Lunch: Spaghetti Squash Pie
Dinner: Beef Stir-Fry with Cauliflower Fried Rice
Dessert: Coconut Cookie Dough

Wednesday

Breakfast: Cauliflower Skillet Casserole
Snack: Peanut Butter Bars
Lunch: Spaghetti Squash Pie
Dinner: Beef Stir-Fry with Cauliflower Fried Rice
Dessert: Coconut Cookie Dough

Thursday

Breakfast: Cauliflower Skillet Casserole
Snack: Peanut Butter Bars
Lunch: Spaghetti Squash Pie
Dinner: Beef Stir-Fry with Cauliflower Fried Rice
Dessert: Coconut Cookie Dough

Friday

Breakfast: Cauliflower Skillet Casserole
Snack: Peanut Butter Bars
Lunch: Spaghetti Squash Pie
Dinner: Beef Stir-Fry with Cauliflower Fried Rice
Dessert: Coconut Cookie Dough

Saturday

Breakfast: Zucchini Latkes (Chapter 17) with 2 poached eggs
Snack: Jalapeño Popper Dip (Chapter 15)
Lunch: Greek Mason Jar Salad (Chapter 8)
Dinner: Supreme Meatza (Chapter 17)
Dessert: Cashew Butter Mousse (Chapter 16)

Sunday

Breakfast: Zucchini Latkes with 2 poached eggs
Snack: Jalapeño Popper Dip
Lunch: Greek Mason Jar Salad
Dinner: Supreme Meatza
Dessert: Cashew Butter Mousse

Shopping List for Two-Week Meal Plan

Produce/Fresh Herbs

16 ounces sliced white mushrooms
4 whole white mushrooms
1 small head green cabbage
2 large red bell peppers
1 large orange bell pepper
1 large green bell pepper
1 small white onion
1 medium yellow onion
1 large spaghetti squash
3 large bulbs garlic (19 cloves)
4 medium jalapeños
3 cups spinach
3 large cucumbers
1 English cucumber
1 large zucchini
2 bunches scallions
2 heads romaine lettuce
4 large heads cauliflower
4 celery stalks
3 medium lemons
1 bunch fresh parsley
1 bunch fresh dill

Meats

1¾ pounds no-sugar-added bacon
2 pounds ground turkey
1 pound ground no-sugar-added turkey sausage
¾ pound ground no-sugar-added chicken sausage
3 pounds ground beef
2 pounds boneless, skinless chicken breasts
½ cup pepperoni (¼ cup chopped)

Dairy/Eggs

3 cups shredded mozzarella cheese
½ cup grated Parmesan cheese
6 tablespoons crumbled feta cheese
2¼ cups shredded Cheddar cheese
24 ounces cream cheese
2½ cups plain Greek yogurt
1 cup heavy whipping cream
3 dozen plus 1 large eggs

Canned Items

5 cans (13.5-ounce) full-fat coconut milk
1 (14-ounce) can chopped artichoke hearts
6 ounces tomato paste
28 ounces no-sugar-added pizza sauce
24 ounces no-sugar-added chicken broth
2 ounces beef broth
½ cup Kalamata olives
¼ cup sliced black olives

Dried Spices/Herbs

3 tablespoons plus ¼ teaspoon salt
4½ teaspoons freshly ground black pepper
2¼ teaspoons onion powder
¾ teaspoon garlic powder
1 teaspoon garlic salt
1 teaspoon dried basil
1½ teaspoons dried oregano
½ teaspoon dried thyme
¼ teaspoon ground sage
1 teaspoon dry mustard powder
¾ teaspoon crushed red pepper flakes
⅛ teaspoon ground cloves
⅛ teaspoon ground allspice
½ teaspoon Chinese five spice

Oil/Vinegar

6 tablespoons olive oil
1 cup plus 2 tablespoons avocado oil
2 tablespoons sesame oil
2 tablespoons apple cider vinegar

Miscellaneous

1½ cups plus 3 tablespoons ghee
4 teaspoons vanilla extract
¼ cup powdered erythritol
½ cup granulated erythritol
⅓ cup unsweetened cacao powder
¼ cup unsweetened shredded coconut
¾ cup coconut flour
1½ cups almond flour
2 teaspoons instant coffee
⅓ cup tahini
½ cup no-sugar-added creamy peanut butter
¼ cup no-sugar-added creamy cashew butter
¼ cup chopped cashews
6 tablespoons coconut aminos
1 teaspoon arrowroot powder
3 tablespoons grass-fed gelatin
2 tablespoons hot chili sauce

Standard US/Metric Measurement Conversions

VOLUME CONVERSIONS

US Volume Measure	Metric Equivalent
⅛ teaspoon	0.5 milliliter
¼ teaspoon	1 milliliter
½ teaspoon	2 milliliters
1 teaspoon	5 milliliters
½ tablespoon	7 milliliters
1 tablespoon (3 teaspoons)	15 milliliters
2 tablespoons (1 fluid ounce)	30 milliliters
¼ cup (4 tablespoons)	60 milliliters
⅓ cup	80 milliliters
½ cup (4 fluid ounces)	125 milliliters
⅔ cup	160 milliliters
¾ cup (6 fluid ounces)	180 milliliters
1 cup (16 tablespoons)	250 milliliters
1 pint (2 cups)	500 milliliters
1 quart (4 cups)	1 liter (about)

WEIGHT CONVERSIONS

US Weight Measure	Metric Equivalent
½ ounce	15 grams
1 ounce	30 grams
2 ounces	60 grams
3 ounces	85 grams
¼ pound (4 ounces)	115 grams
½ pound (8 ounces)	225 grams
¾ pound (12 ounces)	340 grams
1 pound (16 ounces)	454 grams

OVEN TEMPERATURE CONVERSIONS

Degrees Fahrenheit	Degrees Celsius
200 degrees F	95 degrees C
250 degrees F	120 degrees C
275 degrees F	135 degrees C
300 degrees F	150 degrees C
325 degrees F	160 degrees C
350 degrees F	180 degrees C
375 degrees F	190 degrees C
400 degrees F	205 degrees C
425 degrees F	220 degrees C
450 degrees F	230 degrees C

BAKING PAN SIZES

American	Metric
8 × 1½ inch round baking pan	20 × 4 cm cake tin
9 × 1½ inch round baking pan	23 × 3.5 cm cake tin
11 × 7 × 1½ inch baking pan	28 × 18 × 4 cm baking tin
13 × 9 × 2 inch baking pan	30 × 20 × 5 cm baking tin
2 quart rectangular baking dish	30 × 20 × 3 cm baking tin
15 × 10 × 2 inch baking pan	38 × 25 × 5 cm baking tin (Swiss roll tin)
9 inch pie plate	22 × 4 or 23 × 4 cm pie plate
7 or 8 inch springform pan	18 or 20 cm springform or loose bottom cake tin
9 × 5 × 3 inch loaf pan	23 × 13 × 7 cm or 2 lb narrow loaf or pâté tin
1½ quart casserole	1.5 liter casserole
2 quart casserole	2 liter casserole

Index

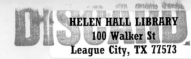